A Mother's Manual For Raising & Recovering Children with Autism

A MOTHER'S MANUAL FOR RAISING AND RECOVERING CHILDREN WITH AUTISM

Published and distributed in the United States by Sonrise Publishing.
Marina Del Rey, California

The author of this book does not dispense medical advice or prescribe the use of any technique as a form of treatment for physical, emotional, or medical problems without the advice of a physician, either directly or indirectly. The intent of the author is only to offer information to help you in your quest for emotional well-being. In the event you use any of the information in this book for yourself, which is your constitutional right, the author and the publisher assume no responsibility for your actions.

First Edition
Self Help

ISBN: 0991434706
ISBN 13: 9780991434701
Library of Congress Control Number: 2014917725
CreateSpace Independent Publishing Platform
North Charleston, South Carolina

A Mother's Manual For Raising & Recovering Children with Autism

Ann Hamiliton Wallace,
MA, MFT, MscD.
and
Jon Wallace

Published by
SONRISE PUBLISHING

Acknowledgements

God, my inspiration and spiritual strength to get through arduous projects.

My husband Larry, and my son, Jon, for sharing me with my creative endeavors and being patient and loving when my mood went south because of self-imposed deadlines.

My friends, who always encourage me to write books.

Marlene Tang, Nina Purtell, and Ansley Allen for generously offering their typing skills.

Reba Merrill for helping the book get to print and teaching me about Amazon e-publishing.

The authors and publishers who gave me permission to use excerpts from their intellectual property.

Thank you so much!
Mark DeAntonio, M.D., for book endorsement
Larry Wallace, for cover photo
Benjamin Wallace
Sue Moffit
Trevor Pacelli
Daniel Hawthorne
David Bessler
Sam Moore
Natasha McBride, M.D.
Jenny McCarthy and Jerry Kartzinel, M.D.

Paige Craig for beautiful interior photos and back cover photos
Nancy Younan Tamer for another superb book cover
Vicki Torres, editing
Esther Gwynne, copy editing

PREFACE

Why write a book like this? There's bound to be intimate details best shared with close friends and family. There's bound to be a lot of work and money spent with no guarantee of compensation. So, why do it?

First, my friends have encouraged me for years to share all the knowledge I amassed raising my Jonnie. They all love him and want others to know how far he's come.

He is truly a "miracle man."

Jon is the joy of all our lives. And he would be your joy too, if you ever met him.

Secondly, I must confess that being an Italian from New York, I have a soft spot in my heart for The Real Housewives of New York and New Jersey. I get a kick out of their accents and mannerisms that remind me of the friends I grew up with. Well, not Teresa (bless her heart!). When I saw Jacqueline Laurita crying on TV—Jacqueline's son has autism—I knew what she was feeling and wished I could share with her the many things I've experienced. I felt frustrated when she said, "These children don't come with a manual; you are in uncharted waters."

Thus, I got the kick in my pants to tell our story. I decided then and there that I would write a manual for mothers and fathers raising children with autism.

To provide a clearer understanding of my story, I have organized this manual by focusing, first, on Jon's remarkable journey. In the first three sections, I recount and relive all the setbacks and triumphs my family experienced.

Next, is the research section. While Jonnie grew up, I was actively searching to find out all I could about treatments and remedies that might help him. Even today, I continue to search for more information. The benefit of all my work is presented in that section. It represents key knowledge I found that gave me hope and helped me during his recovery.

The summation is a celebration, as is, truthfully, the entire book.

TABLE OF CONTENTS

SECTION I

EARLY YEARS

CHAPTER 1

Conceiving

Today is a big day. Today I take the first step toward recounting the joys and hardships of our autistic journey. It's the first time I will have a co-author, my son, Jon. No illusions here; we will struggle to agree on the important issues and probably a lot of other things. In the end, the finished product will be entertaining, educational, and uniquely our own. A lot of sweat, tears and laughter will be shared, but I predict all will turn out right.

It's about now I am wondering why I didn't keep a daily journal. Everything would be so much easier. Easier is something that is not in my astrological chart. As a matter of fact, I was told years ago that my chart was a tyrant. I was told I would have many obstacles to overcome and definitely warned not to have another child. Life has a funny way of playing tricks on you. The more you resist something, the more it persists. Another child was always in the back of my mind.

Around the time my daughter, my firstborn, was 15 years old and fiercely independent, my husband and I started actively trying to have another baby. Trying to conceive at 37 years old with a husband who has had a vasectomy meant many, many doctor visits, blood draws, surgery, and disappointments. Finally, after three years, we became pregnant. Four months later, I miscarried and cried a river in the backyard. I told my husband, "That's it! I give up; no more!" I remembered the astrologer's admonition ("Don't have another child."). My husband, Larry, knew how much I wanted another baby and how brokenhearted I was. He convinced me to try just one more month to see if we could succeed. The stars in the heaven aligned just right to make a wish come true. At 40 years old, I had conceived for the second time. To me, this was my miracle child. The doctor insisted on an amniocentesis. The procedure revealed a healthy baby boy was in our future.

As my belly grew, I was intensely studying to obtain my Marriage, Family and Child Certification. Every day, another chapter to commit to memory. The childhood disorders were the hardest to cope with. I would tremble a bit when reading about childhood schizophrenia or pervasive developmental disorder. Surely I could relax, I thought; all the children in our family tree were healthy. But remember, what you resist persists. I worried about being 40 and everything else that comes with it. I tried to avoid being neurotic while I was studying so hard and carrying a baby. Being pregnant was not a walk in the park for me. I endured migraines without even a Tylenol®. I developed a terrible pain in my side so severe I ended up in the hospital. My gynecologist wanted to sedate me to explore the problem. I argued with him: wait a day or two to avoid anesthesia. He wouldn't relent, so I changed doctors during the middle of my distress. A friend recommended her doctor and called him to see me in the hospital. We waited a couple of days and the pain subsided. Thank God! If I had agreed to anesthesia while pregnant, I can't imagine the guilt I would have had to endure.

Walking became harder and harder as each day passed. The baby's head was positioned low in my pelvis. My supervisor at the Adolescent Rehab Unit where I worked suggested I stay home with my feet up. Before I could break away from and say goodbye to the kids for whom I cared so much, I came down with a nasty virus. That convinced me I had to take care of myself immediately. I scheduled a C-section 10 days before my due date because of the severe pelvic pain, and I asked Larry to take me to the Chart House restaurant on Pacific Coast Highway for a slice of mud pie. I realized something as decadent as that gooey chocolate and coffee concoction would not be practical after the baby was born!

Even with many advances in pain meds since my first C-section, I had a hard time. I have fibromyalgia, an overabundance of substance P in my spinal fluid, which makes me extremely sensitive to pain. I begged the doctor and nurse to leave my morphine drip for one more day. The nurse tried to persuade my husband that I was becoming an addict and suggested taking me off all pain medications immediately. I screamed and threw both of them out of my room. This was the beginning of a long journey with emotional challenges and miraculous happenings.

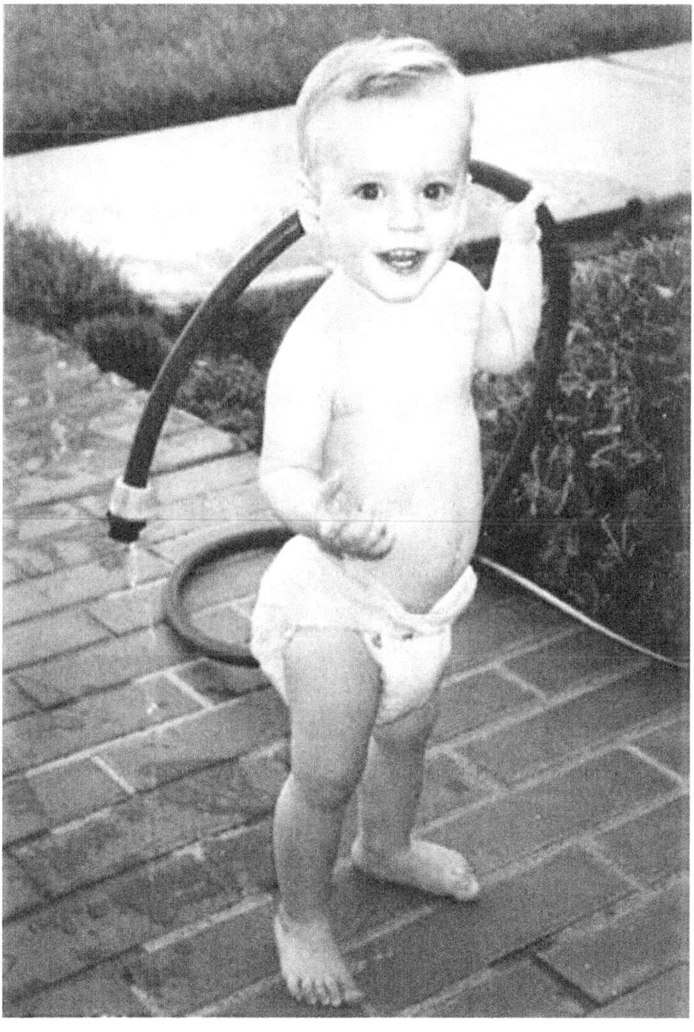

JON CIRCA 1 YEAR OLD

CHAPTER 2

Early Stirrings of Problems to Come

Jon Thomas Wallace came into this world on June 28, 1989. He was the most beautiful boy I ever saw: white-blond hair, blue eyes that could pull you into his world, 7 pounds 11 ounces, and 21-inches long with an Apgar (newborn health) score of 10. A perfect score for my little bundle of joy! But two days into our hospital stay, Jon began to look yellow. We found out he had high levels of bilirubin, a chemical produced by the body and normally excreted through urine. Therefore, when we arrived at home we had bili lights with us. These lights break down bilirubin and return the levels to the normal range. As I would glance into the nursery, my little treasure was curled up on his lamb's wool cover and lit as though he was a work of art. Soon thereafter, the lights were no longer needed and life became normal. We hired a night nurse, Carmen, to help the first month. She was desperately needed because of my recovery from the C-section and I was still studying for my oral examination.

It so happened I had two good friends who delivered babies at the same time. This was helpful; we exchanged stories and advice among us. The only problem was their children were hitting milestones before Jon. At three months, their babies were sleeping through the night. Jon was not. The other babies were babbling and saying "mamma" and "dada." Jon did not.

To make matters worse, Jon would cry off and on for 24 hours a day. Everyone took turns walking him and rocking him. This included a live-in housekeeper that became a necessity. My daughter, Danielle, became overwhelmed with the care process and started looking at alternative living arrangements. I am sure she also believed that we were just spoiling him. Spoiling a mid-life child is not uncommon. After all, most parents have more time, money, and patience than they had in their 20's with their first children. Even though we were better equipped to raise this child, I didn't believe spoiling children was in their best interest. Still, life as we knew it had ended. The Wallace household definitely revolved around Jon. I thought that was OK. For the first three years, I even convinced myself that it was desirable. What was not normal was the fact that Jon was not sleeping through the night yet. Other babies had been blabbering for some time and my darling had just started speaking at 2 ½ years old. Our pediatrician was concerned about Jon's delay in speech, but he assured us that 2 ½ years old was the benchmark for speech to begin and Jon made that milestone on the cusp of normal.

As we inched into our fourth year and a good night's sleep remained elusive, I began to become anxious when I climbed into my bed at night. Something had to be done. We took Jon to a specialist to address his large tonsils that caused him some distress at night. The doctor promptly recommended removing them as a way to perhaps help Jon sleep through the night. From the moment we came home from the hospital, Jon breathed so much better. A few times we even went into the nursery to check on him because his labored breathing had disappeared and the nursery monitor was silent. Unfortunately, however, the surgery did not make Jon sleep through the night. What to do? I researched sleep problems and came up with the Ferber method. Created by Dr. Richard Ferber, former director of the Center for Pediatric Sleep Disorders at Boston Children's Hospital, the method involves training your child to self soothe by allowing the child to cry for short amounts of time, maybe three minutes, before receiving external comfort from the parent.

Everything sounds easier than it is, but it worked. After spending a few evenings on the outside of Jon's door crying because *he* was crying, our baby began to comfort himself. Within a week of employing the technique, Jon was sleeping through the night.

I was so happy, everything was great. Jon was speaking and sleeping appropriately, life was good. Only one problem persisted. Every time we wanted to take Jon to a restaurant or shopping mall, he screamed. His screams would continue until we returned to our home and his familiar surroundings. Later, I understood these outings were just too stimulating for our little boy. So, everything became routine. We would leave Jon home when we had to get out of the house for a while. When we returned, Jon would be lining up all his stuffed animals along the playroom walls. I thought this behavior was enchanting. Sometimes ignorance is bliss. After all, he was walking, talking, and toileting with the best of them. As a matter of fact, he was agile and strong in the "kids' gym."

CHAPTER 3

Northridge Earthquake and Emma

The Northridge earthquake on Jan. 17, 1994, devastated our home. Fortunately, our house withstood the shaking, but the asbestos was disturbed. All the ductwork for heating and air needed replacing; ceilings needed scraping. Our family moved out and lived in the Marriott hotel for a month. Imagine the disruption for our child, for whom leaving the home for even a few hours created major stress for him and us. To make matters worse, the cleaning people threw Jon's "security blanket" into the general laundry never to be found again. Then, the insurance company wanted us to move again. Unwilling to pay for the hotel and meals, they suggested moving yet again, this time to a townhouse nearby while the renovations dragged on and on. In the midst of all the confusion I was actively looking for a new housekeeper and nanny for Jon. I can't remember how I found Emma. Perhaps I ran an ad and she replied. I interviewed several people and decided on this young woman after calling her reference. Emma's reference answered the phone and was very generous with her time. She explained that Emma had worked for her a few months earlier and she loved how Emma cared for her four children. The woman said she bought Emma many gifts to show her appreciation, even robes and towels monogrammed with Emma's name on them to make her feel special. But, without warning, one day Emma announced she was leaving. The woman said her eyes filled with tears as they parted. I thought perhaps taking care of four children was just too much for a young girl. I made excuses for this abrupt, unusual behavior.

I decided to hire Emma and give her a chance. From the beginning, she was very good at organizing the new household and caring for Jon. I thought, "This is too good to be true!"

Usually it takes a month or so to train someone and for them to make the transition.

I thought things were going smoothly. I took a chance to exhale. Typically, when I hire someone, I make them promise as a hiring requirement that they stay for a year and give me a month's notice if they have to end employment. I try to avoid too much change in Jon's life. I don't think change is in his best interest.

Emma slept in Jon's room at the townhouse. The insurance company paid for a two-bedroom, two-bath unit. They were each in their own twin bed. At night, I felt like I had two kids, so when I kissed Jon goodnight, I kissed Emma, too!

Everything was seemingly going well. Oh, happy day! We fell into a routine after two or three months in which my husband, Larry, drove Emma to the bus stop so she could go home on the weekends. We would pick her up on Monday.

But unbeknownst to me, Emma was already scheming her way out of her agreement with me and finding excuses to leave, sometimes using outright lies. One Friday afternoon as Larry drove her to the bus stop, she told him she wouldn't be coming back. Jon had bitten her, she said, which I knew was a lie because she had never mentioned it to me. When I asked Jonnie, he started crying, promising me she was lying. Then the biggest lie of all. She "confided in Larry" that on one occasion I had been mean to her. Larry didn't know what to make of it. He couldn't believe it. Emma said I had yelled at her and accused her of using my makeup, which she vehemently denied. As if I would be upset and yell over such a minor action! But, Emma insisted, for these reasons, she would not be returning Monday. She was gone, likely spreading rumors, failing to give notice so that I had time to replace her, and breaking her verbal contract to stay one year! Any child would have suffered from such behavior, but for Jonnie, it was even tougher.

CHAPTER 4

The Discovered Journal

Although I began this book lamenting that I had failed to keep a journal, I made an unexpected and happy discovery. As I gathered records and information to supplement this book, I came across an attempt at journaling—about two weeks of efforts total. When I read these new-found pages, I couldn't believe how difficult those times were!

So, I offer this intimate view into our lives at the beginning of our journey. If you are struggling with an autistic child or one with learning disabilities, I wish my notes will inspire you to hope in copious amounts, when you finally see how far we have come.

Jon was 5 years old when I wrote these notes and we were just at the beginning of our journey. Many things slowly improved over the years. Steadily, I got my son back and recovered the wonderful young man he is today, something I couldn't have known in 1994.

August 1994

Today I hired a new housekeeper and nanny for Jon. She is bright and friendly. I'm afraid she won't stay if Jon continues to "act out." For the first time today, Jon engaged in self- injurious behavior. I was horrified! I called Dr. Bebe. I told him to prescribe something to calm Jon down. I told Dr. Bebe, Emma and I needed some pills too (ha-ha). Emma cried when she saw Jon so upset, he was biting his arm and pulling his hair. I know from current research that this happens when a child is reaching toxic overload.

According to Dr. Jerry Kartzinel, Autism = toxic overload! Toxic overload leads to regression. Dr. Jerry Kartzinel: "There are two forms of regression. The first, more obvious one, is the loss of a particular skill or skills. The second form of regression is not acquiring a particular trait in the same time period as his neurotypical peers are. It's a failure to keep up with his peers. Children with autism have a tendency to develop stereotypical repetitive behaviors (stimming), like moving their arms, their hands, flapping, odd movements and gestures. They do not develop normal toy play. They become very repetitive and then they can be very obsessive-compulsive, perseverative, and anxious."

Dr. Bebe said, "Often by the time you drive to the pharmacy the tantrum will be over." He was right. I'm still glad I have the medication: It gives me some sort of security.

Jon went for his five-year checkup. He endured many booster shots and a barrage of tests. Dr. McLaren (Jon's pediatrician at the time) said he agrees with Dr. Gabriel (a neurologist) that Jon is not autistic. Today I received Gabriel's report, most of it I can't understand. Dr. Gabriel believes Jon is developmentally behind, but will catch up. "Jon's not autistic."

Another day in August 1994

Jon continues to be more agitated than usual lately. It could be the presence of Emma or the absence and reappearance of his father. This time Larry was away 10 days in Africa. Jon also fell while walking on a slippery curb. He nearly impaled himself on a tall sprinkler head.

Jon is learning to swim. We have a very kind woman teaching him. She's warm and loving and knows just how to handle him. Today he took his first few strokes in the pool by himself.

Sonnie's BBQ

We went to Sonnie's BBQ today. Jon played soccer with the "big boys." He did real well with all the new people.

Rosalee, a best friend of Sonnie's, observed Jon in the backyard and then observed, "Don't worry about that boy; he's not autistic. I'm in education and I know."

The experts at UCLA say Jon is autistic. Dr. Gabriel, some friends, and family members say no, he's not. It's like watching a tennis match back and forth. He is, he isn't, he is, he isn't.

It's hard not to worry when your child can't remember how old he is and is scheduled for hospitalization next week.

Early August 1994

Jon was agitated when he returned from school. Dad gave him a three-minute "time out" on the patio.

My mother called to tell me Sally Jesse Raphael's TV show today was called "Autism and Children." Tomorrow, I will try to track down that videotape. Jon was playing a lot with his paper airplanes. Suddenly, he began kissing me and Emma doggy style. I told him that only husbands and wives could kiss that way. He is becoming a little Casanova.

August 13, 1994

Jon started licking his dad today. Larry said that was nasty. Jon continued. When I told Jon he could pick up bacteria that way, he stopped.

Today I read a letter from the office of U.S. District Court Judge Sam C. Pointer, who in 1994 oversaw a class-action breast implant liability case. The letter mentioned the possibility of children being affected by silicone implants in utero or from breast milk. I knew this before they ever dreamed of admitting it!

Today Jon said he wanted to marry all the girls in town. So, Larry pointed to the *TV Guide* cover with three beauties in bathing suits, the girls from the TV show, *Bay Watch*. Jon thought for a moment and said, "They already have a man." A man was posed on the cover with the women. Jon is so cute sometimes and smart when he wants to be!

August 21, 1994

Tomorrow we go to the hospital again. I don't know if we will be there for 24 hours or five days. I'm packing with lots of help from Jon while Larry begs Jon for some respite, asking him to stop tearing his shirt. But all and all, Jon's been good this weekend.

August 23, 1994

Last night I did not sleep a wink. The hospital staff kept coming in and turning on the bright light above our heads. Someday, I hope this child will know how much I loved him. Somehow Jon was able to sleep through it all, strange! Jon looks like a little Smurf, in his telemetry cap. Larry took some photos. Finally, the doctors have induced seizures in me. No sleep, no coffee, no lunch for Jon, that's it. I think I feel one coming on right now. Our ordeal lasted three days and three nights. The doctors found spikes in Jon's sleep cycle one night. I guess that means he is three times more likely to develop seizures in his lifetime.

Saturday, November 5, 1994—Ritalin Trials

We gave Jon one 5 mg tablet at about 9:00 a.m. He was doing great all morning, nice and calm. But then, he was already calm before we gave him the medication this morning. About noon, Jon had a rebound and acted out terribly in the restaurant. We gave him another 5 mg about 1 p.m. He was OK after that at lunch. We couldn't decide if the improvement was the meds or lunch.

November 11, 1994

Sunday was a repeat of Saturday. Monday I sent Jon to school with a letter to his teacher, Mrs. Renfield, and Mrs. Fajnor, the resource teacher. I explained to them about the Ritalin trial and asked them to observe him this week to access his ability to concentrate.

Mrs. Fajnor reported to me that she saw no difference. His counselor, Cindy at the WVJCC, said he was rebounding a lot in the afternoons. He was agitated and becoming aggressive with some of the kids. I noticed he began bed-wetting all this week.

I called Dr. Bebe and told him about Jon's agitation and bed-wetting. He suggested doubling the dose!

Friday was Veterans' Day and a great opportunity for me to observe Jon all day and make a final decision about continuing the medication. In the morning, I asked Jon if he liked his Ritalin pill. He said no. I asked if he felt nervous and he said yes. I gave him the morning dose hesitantly and began drilling him about his letters. His lesson went well.

We left for McDonald's and I gave him an overlapping dose to test Dr. Bebe's suggestion. Jon regressed and could not make eye contact with some little friends who stopped by our table to say hello. "That's it," I said to myself. He looks like he took a giant step backward, circa 3 years old.

We went to get a haircut right after McDonald's.

Jon was miserable meeting this new person, could not make eye contact, and forgot how old he was. I felt so guilty for giving him the second Ritalin after only two hours from the first one.

It was clear to me: NO MORE.

Sunday I start the DMG suggested by Dr. Rimland.

<u>November, 15, 1994</u>

Today I found a lady to help me clean the townhouse. I thought life was beginning to get under control, even though my back (slipped disc) was not responding to physical therapy, as I had hoped it would. I arrived at Jon's afternoon program to find him in the director's office. I was told Jon had been exposing himself and cursing out of control. Thank God he is only 5 years old! Time out did not work either. The supervisor asked me if something could be done. I said I didn't know.

I left there feeling so low the sidewalk looked like up to me. I came home and I regressed to calling my mother. She came over and began yelling at me for being so upset. I really needed a break. Is this when children are sent away? What a thought! My life could be so good, but someone must be cursing me.

That's all I wrote from that period and have shared with you: two weeks in the life of a mother raising a child with what she suspected was autism, 1994.

CHAPTER 5

Preschool and Elementary School

When Jon first entered preschool, it became a running joke that I could always be found camped outside his classroom door. The process was that all mothers were invited to join the class the first day; then we were expected to leave the kids and go home. I knew my Jonnie was sensitive, so I sat in the hallway a good part of the first month. I would ease my way down the hallway and out to the parking lot. When finally, Jon was not appearing in the hallway looking for Mommy anymore, the transition was made. I realized this was becoming a pattern. Jon would adjust to new situations eventually, but it took him much longer than other kids.

Preschool at St. Luke's gave way to a year of preschool at Meadow Oaks, a highly regarded school in the Calabasas countryside. It was a dramatic contrast. Jon's first preschool was very small with teachers who acted more like mothers than disciplinarians. Meadow Oaks school was posh and the mothers had agonizingly high standards, even in preschool. The large campus bustled with excitement and adventures. Even though I knew Jon needed to move into a less sequestered environment, he would have some difficult days ahead. At Meadow Oaks, there was no fudging around with the rules. Mothers met the teachers, saw the classroom, and left for the day. Heart in hand, I followed the protocol, hoping Jon would make the transition. The only reason I agreed to leave when I did was the beautiful smile on the face of his teacher, Mrs. Gilley. I am usually a good judge of character, and by my observations, she was delightful and competent.

Jon didn't cry when I left him at Meadow Oaks, so I assumed all was well. After some time, Mrs. Gilley asked if I could come into school for a parent/teacher conference. I was eager to get an update on Jon's progress. Mrs. Gilley explained that Jon had a best friend named Jamison. I thought, "Oh that's great." And I was happy that they bonded. The only drawback was that both boys were not adjusting well to the classroom environment.

Jamison was the tallest in the class and Jon was the shortest, which made for a comical odd couple. Jamison was hyperactive and could not sit still for more than 10 minutes; Jon would sit under his desk for as long as Mrs. Gilley allowed him. The teacher's hands were full with teaching advanced curriculum to the general population, while constantly seating Jamison and trying to get Jon to focus on the material. I thanked Jon's teacher for all the attention she gave him, and assured her I was not worried about the numbers and letters. I expected Jon would catch up in kindergarten. I believed he was getting a valuable experience just being away from Mom and being in a somewhat chaotic situation. I was sure his year at Meadow Oaks better prepared Jon to adjust to his next year at public school.

The public school for our neighborhood was Woodland Hills Elementary. They prided themselves on teaching gifted children and not having special education on their campus. Every school has its favorite teachers and most parents jockeyed for the best instructor for their kids. In short order, I figured out that none of the parents wanted Mrs. Renfield. I checked the board and my heart sank. Jon had been assigned to Renfield's class. I heard parents actually crying when they got the same news. Knowing my Jonnie still needed special attention to focus on his schoolwork, I promptly set up an appointment to see the principal. I explained my concerns and requested the other kindergarten teacher, whom I had heard was kind and knowledgeable. The principal brushed me off. "That's ridiculous. Mrs. Renfield is a great teacher, just give her a chance," he said.

Most of the time I *do* believe mother knows best. I now advise moms not to be bullied or dissuaded by "authority figures," but to hold fast and always do what's in the best interest of the child. I learned this the hard way by letting Mrs. Renfield have a chance. She didn't seem to notice what I quickly discovered for myself by watching him in the classroom. It's a custom in most kindergarten classes to have two mothers volunteer to help out with the class. I participated with the other moms in this weekly ritual. I had a bird's eye view of how Jon was adjusting and how his learning style compared to the others. I could see Jon was still immature compared to his peers. I thought it might be time for a professional evaluation.

CHAPTER 6

Diagnosis and Failure to Thrive

Diagnosis

I chose B.J. Freeman, PhD., a past director of the UCLA Autism Evaluation Clinic and an expert on neurological disorders and autism. At the time of our visit to B.J., I was licensed in the State of California as a Marriage, Family, and Child therapist. So I knew something about autism. But Jon did not fit the profile I had in my head. He was speaking and he did not bang his head or toe walk. Also, he seemed to form attachments to some of his playmates. But I knew he was different from the daughter I raised and from his other peers. Jon was slightly delayed and immature for his age. He was also very small for his age. He hadn't gained weight for three years and remained at 35 pounds and in a car seat forever. Before he entered public school, I had been told that holding him back a year and starting him in kindergarten the next year would be best. This was the first time I advocated strongly for Jon. Absolutely not! Whatever was troubling Jon would not be fixed by another year of kindergarten. If Jon needed extra help to focus, we would get him a tutor. I didn't want all of his friends to go on to first grade and leave him behind.

So, having seen for myself how Jon struggled in kindergarten, I was glad to have found an expert. When Dr. Freeman entered the room, I could tell by her demeanor she was going to tell us what was up with Jon. I didn't have any doubts about that. As she led Jon away to the examination room I whispered in her ear, "Can a child be a little autistic?"

"We will talk about that later," was all she said.

Larry and I watched hopefully as B.J. put Jon through a plethora of tests. I thought he was amazingly brave following directions like a little soldier with this stranger. After two or three hours we were ushered into B.J.'s office for her educated opinion.

"I'm sorry to have to tell you this, but I believe Jon has autism," she told us. "Do you see on these tests how he scored so high in some areas and very low on others? This is an indication of autism. And no, Mrs. Wallace a child cannot be a little autistic. It's like being pregnant, you are or you aren't."

The news hit me like a punch in the stomach. I stood in disbelief not knowing what to do next. I was paralyzed with fear and couldn't make the conscious decision to even move my legs. Thank God, B.J. had orders in her hand for a telemetry exam the following week at UCLA. This exam would tell us if Jon was having seizures or was prone to seizures. Autistic children can have a propensity toward seizures, and it's a good idea to find out as soon as possible. Now that we had a focus—the test—I was able to gather my senses and leave her office in a dignified manner.

It became clear to me on the ride home that I needed to get up to speed with the latest research regarding my son's condition. This little-known condition that used to rear its ugly head in one in 10,000 individuals was escalating into a modern-day epidemic. The statistics were staggering. One in 1,000, became one in 500, became one in 250, became one in 150! I couldn't believe my ears when I heard about the sharp increase in cases at the time of Jon's diagnosis. I wanted to understand why. I thought this was the purpose to which I could dedicate my life. With renewed vigor, my husband and I plunged into the reality of full-time caregivers and research specialists.

Soon, my family was camped out at UCLA Hospital. Jon's brain was wired up to numerous electrodes that recorded his EEG waves continuously for three days. They challenged him with strobe lights to see if the lights would induce a seizure. It was difficult to see my baby hooked up to machines and confined to a bed. For an active boy, that alone was a nightmare. As a family, we were prepared to do whatever was necessary to help our son. . Thankfully, the news was fantastic. No seizures were recorded. I thought to myself, "It is important to get an expert to be straight with you and advise you about relevant tests to be done."

Today, I always recommend finding the best doctor possible that treats autism. Be sure to rule out seizures from the beginning. If you had a heart problem you wouldn't go to a dermatologist. So, if you have any suspicion your child is struggling, you must enlist a pediatric neurologist or autism specialist. Never, never, never put your head in the sand and ignore speech delays and developmental issues. The sooner the child is diagnosed, the better the prognosis will be. The best treatment starts at around 3 years old. Jonnie didn't get diagnosed until five. I felt very bad about that. But I vowed to do my very best from that time on. I promised myself to be hyper vigilant and not let any grass grow under my feet.

Failure to Thrive

As important as the autism diagnosis was, of nearly equal importance was treatment for failure to thrive, a medical condition seen in children. Observing Jon with his peers at kindergarten, I became keenly aware of the size differential that existed. Most children his age were wearing size 5 or 6X and were out of their car seats. Jonnie was in a 2T, weighed 35 pounds, and had to be strapped into his car seat. I had learned my lesson; no time to waste, off to the pediatric endocrinologist. Thank you God, my husband had excellent health insurance through his work. It was like déjà vu and in no time we were back at the hospital. Poor little Jon had to have insulin injections to test his growth hormone. It's the only way to get an accurate reading. The child must be in the hospital and carefully monitored. The results came back and he was in the normal range. Growth hormone treatment is very expensive and insurance companies often will discourage starting a regimen. Just recently, Kaiser Permanente tried to scare my dear friend from using GH by citing very rare side effects.

They kept telling my friend to wait and see how her son grew. Now they admit his growth spurt has ended at 5′ 4″ tall. They say growth hormone at this stage may give him a chance to reach 5′ 6″. I reassured my girlfriend that her son is so personable and smart, he will do well even if he is 5′ 6″ or less. In the case of my son, he already had a mighty challenge to contend with. I was not going to permit him to be challenged by height as well. I fought hard with second opinions and justified my cause with facts. Jon was in the 75th percentile at birth; but he was 15% below the growth chart. His parents were in the 75th percentile and that's what I wanted for him. With persistence, the insurance company relented and decided to do a trial run. Jon responded to the trial so well, he was permitted to continue his treatment until age 17. Jon is now 6′ 2″ tall and wows the crowds when he passes by. Jon went with me to one of my doctors last year and the doctor could not stop calling him Apollo. Jon chuckled and sometimes I call him Apollo, also.

When I decided to write this book, I couldn't decide on the best title. My first choice was *Canaries in the Coal Mine* or *My Life as a Lioness*. The reason was that as a child I was raised to be seen and not heard. This made me painfully shy and, according to my father, too sensitive. Having Jon made me emerge from a scaredy cat to a ferocious lioness.

When it came to Jon's care, there weren't any lengths I wouldn't go to or battles I would not fight. You didn't mess with him or momma lion could bite your head off. Also, along the way I marveled at how brave, cunning and ferocious my little cub was becoming. He would need every advantage possible to deal with challenges and obstacles along the way, as well as people unwilling to help him.

CHAPTER 7

Elementary School—Run!

This brings me back to his kindergarten teacher, Mrs. Renfield. As soon as Jon was diagnosed, I found a simple, easy-to-read book on the subject to share with his teacher.

I mistakenly thought that by knowing Jon had autism, she would realize his daydreaming was not intentional. I also wholeheartedly believed any teacher having care of my child for the better part of the day must know what his special needs are. I found out later she scoffed at the book and told her assistant she had no intention of taking on any extra burdens when it came to Jon.

Soon, I was introduced to Mrs. Fajnor, the resource teacher. Remember, no special education classes existed at Jon's "hip" school. Arlene Fajnor was a no-nonsense veteran teacher who had been around the block a few times. She knew her stuff and, even though she could be intimidating at first, always had the best interest of children in her heart. The first thing she said to me was, "Stop carrying that child around like a baby. Put him down!"

I had become so accustomed to walking with Jonnie on my hipbone, I actually ruptured a disc. Even though he was 5 years old he looked like 2 ½, and when he said, "Mommy carry me," I was only too happy to oblige. I could see she started sizing up Jon's needs from that very minute. I didn't care that she was not trying to win a popularity contest with me. Mrs. Fajnor became the happiest part of Jon's first year at Woodland Hills Elementary. Later she would become a dear family friend and tutor to Jon.

Jon would walk from his homeroom class to Mrs. Fajnor's resource class every day. He would have to walk a long way across the campus by himself. Oh, wait a minute. "By himself? No way!"

"What if he wandered out into the neighborhood on his own?" I objected. So, Jon was escorted to resource for several weeks until he became so familiar with the routine he was safe to go on his own. By the middle of the year, I thought maybe all was well. But in the back of my mind, I knew his teacher, Mrs. Renfield, was not liked by most parents and there had to be a reason for that.

I soon discovered a reason to feel the same. One of the mothers with whom I became friendly and who volunteered in the classroom observed Mrs. Renfield treating Jon like a dog. Marlene Tang is a soft-spoken, lovely person who gets along with everyone. She is not the type to rock the boat or cause controversy. So, when she told me she couldn't take seeing the poor treatment, I believed every word she said. As it happened, the very next day Jon was in the principal's office in tears over an incident in Renfield's class. As part of his physical therapy for a weak handgrip, Jon squeezed a spray bottle of water several times a day to increase the strength in his hands. But Mrs. Renfield had a spray bottle with chemicals on her desk and left the room. When Jon spotted saw the bottle on the teacher's desk, he grabbed it and began showing his classmates how he practiced every day. Upon her return, Mrs. Renfield chastised Jon severely and sent him to the principal for endangering his classmates by spewing chemicals into the air.

I was livid. Why did she leave a bottle of chemicals unattended when she left the room, herself endangering students? Instead, she refused to accept responsibility and blamed an autistic child. How despicable! Outraged, I gave the principal my opinion of her behavior, plus, shared the information I had received from Marlene. I demanded Jon be transferred to the teacher of my choice for the rest of the year. I was not soft-spoken or kind; I was enraged that I had allowed the principal to persuade me to accept a poor teacher who harmed my son. We got a wonderful teacher to finish the school year.

That's why I now advise mothers and fathers to never allow themselves to be talked out of what's in the best interest of their children. School officials will give excuses such as, "That class is full," or "We don't have money in the budget to support that service."

Be shameless; be brave as the lion in defense of your son or daughter. Their welfare should be your only concern. Raising special needs children is not for the weak of heart. You will need support and perhaps even therapy along the way. Please get it. Not only for yourself, but for your child's future. A healthy, emotionally strong parent is needed on this journey from childhood to adulthood especially if you and your child are going to survive and prosper in this process.

Hillary Clinton said, "It takes a village to raise a child," and it is especially so for children with special needs. The more help you can amass, the better you will weather the storms ahead. Don't be falsely prideful about asking for favors from your friends and family. If you are married and want a chance for your marriage to survive, take care of yourself, too. Divorce statistics have shown that about 50% of marriages end up failing. For marriages with special needs children, it is almost 100%. Be aware of this pitfall and take care of each other. Nothing could be sadder than ending up in divorce facing all of the challenges ahead alone. Also, your child will have another trauma to contend with on their road to recovery.

So, I always say get that hot tub you've been talking about and use it often. Ask a relative or respite worker to spend the night. Go to the bed-and-breakfast at the beach with your loved one. You know what I am talking about!

By the time we finished our first year at Woodland Hills Elementary, I was ready to pull Jon and run from the school. I could see that they only tolerated him. Our pastor, Joel Osteen, has preached in a sermon, "Do not go where you are tolerated, go where you are celebrated."

I was ready.

CHAPTER 8

Selecting The Right School

We found a school in Tarzana, just one town away, that had an exceptional special education teacher. Mrs. Hurley turned out to be a treasure. Everything about Wilbur School was lovely. You could feel the warmth from everyone you met, from the secretaries at the front desk to the principal, nurse, and our lunchroom monitor, Miss Hattie Brown. Hattie Brown was a large woman with a heart to match her size. No one messed with her, so when she said, "Line up!" or anything else, the children listened. Jon was still so small for his age; I immediately enlisted her help to keep a special eye on him in the lunch line or recess. If you were nearby you could hear Miss Hattie Brown calling Jon to her side, "Come here my baby, come stay with Hattie Brown." I loved that woman!

Jon's classroom consisted of Mrs. Hurley and her assistant, Mrs. Cohen, with eight children and two personal aides for children with problems focusing. The aides, called "shadows," stay close to the children and tap them on the shoulder when they notice their minds wandering. They present some classroom materials to the child in a way that best suits their learning differences. For example, Mrs. Hurley may be speaking to the class on a subject. The aide would present the same concepts visually for visual learners or tactically for kinesthetic learners. This creates individualized learning with an IEP (Individual Education Program) for a superior, special education.

Do not make the mistake of feeling embarrassed about "special education." It's just what it is purported to be, and that's special. All classes and teachers are not equal, so do your homework and choose the best fit for your child.

Do not let school put your child in any class that you feel isn't the best fit for your son or daughter. They will sometimes badger you about placement, so hold your ground. If necessary, hire an advocate familiar with getting your child's type of needs met. The school district must by law provide you with a list of your rights. They must include a list of advocates, lawyers, and appeals processes. Make good use of any resources available to you, because your child is worth it.

The earlier your child gets special attention, the better the outcome. In Jon's case, his education was fantastic. His teacher prepared him well. After three years, Jon caught up to his peers and was ready to mainstream into the fourth grade. But, along the way, a couple of hiccups occurred. The first: Mrs. Hurley suggested I feed Jonnie a few small teaspoons of peanut butter to fatten him up. I got out a little silver baby spoon and filled it with my best organic peanut butter. Into his little mouth it went without any fuss. Jon seemed to like it.

"Great, I'll just give him one more spoonful," I thought. Down the hatch it went. Suddenly, within a few minutes, his eyes were red and swollen; his body covered in hives. I put him immediately in an oatmeal bath and gave him some Benadryl. Then I remembered that some allergies could be life threatening. I called the paramedics. The ambulance arrived and took Jon swiftly to the hospital. On the way, the paramedics gave Jon an epinephrine shot. Thus began some mighty worries about Jon's safety. He would have to be super careful and read labels whenever he ate baked goods or ate in restaurants. I would have to carry EpiPens in case of slipups, and there were a few. Jamming that thick needle into his thigh was not pleasant. The alternative? He might stop breathing. That always overcame any hesitation I had.

"God doesn't give you more than you can handle," I thought, but I began telling Him I was at the precipice of falling apart.

My husband worked very hard to be the sole support of the family. This allowed me to focus all my attention on Jon. Sometimes, Larry would be gone more than he was home. One year, three movies caused him to be away for almost the entire year. I really had to toughen up and move forward, even though I was challenged to my max. I had to handle emergency visits to the hospital and squabbles at school. By this time the shy, quiet kitten had become a ferocious lioness. I had become a no-nonsense woman. I didn't have time for adults behaving badly. I avoided toxic people like the plague. Anything that took my focus off Jon was actively avoided.

The second hiccup that occurred at Wilbur School was Michael and James. These boys were strong and very, very tall. Jon came up to their mid chest. Boys will be boys. One day the cajoling and messing around with Jon went too far. One of them started to choke Jon. Jon was tiny but mighty and with a quick wit. Perhaps, I forgot to mention that. B.J. [Dr. Freeman] told us Jon was very smart. He just couldn't access certain abilities because of his learning differences. Thus, special ed. In a flash, Jon figured out he was in danger. He promptly bit his way out of a tough situation.

This brought a meeting with his teacher the next day. Mrs. Hurley explained that the children were not allowed to be physical with each other and that two wrongs did not make a right. I replied that Jon was simply defending himself, did not start the fight, and that his solution was brilliant. I told her I would encourage him to use the maneuver whenever he feels himself in danger. The conversation ended. I wouldn't give an inch. By now this had become my M.O. in defense of my son. I fully understood and lived the saying, "When the going gets tough, the tough get going."

CHAPTER 9

Exercise, Horse Riding, Master Lee, And Tae Kwan Do

Tae Kwon Do

In one area, however, I didn't need to be tough for Jon. Karate was his to command. Jon was tiny but mighty, and definitely had a fighting spirit. This spirit would not only serve him well in karate but in overcoming obstacles in his future.

By this time, Jon had long ago stopped screaming day and night and had become quite charming, at least outside of home. Sometimes when he came home, mighty meltdowns would erupt. I understood; he needed a safe place to vent his frustrations. Jon had to work a thousand times harder than other children to survive the overstimulation of our times. He had to strain his brain to process information as fast as his peers. These processing problems would persist even into adulthood.

But in karate, Master Lee succumbed to Jon's charms and soon Jon was the teacher's pet. Jon was kinesthetically superior to most others with a gorgeous body sculpted to perfection. His agility and abilities were off the charts. Jon stayed with Master Lee for 10 years. He earned a 4th Dan Black Belt, a ranking of skills unheard of for such a youngster. He was now a master of Tae Kwon Do. Later, his hard work would pay off. Master Lee was never told that Jon was autistic and he didn't teach him any differently than his other students. Jon remembered and picked up everything very quickly! No special concessions were made because no special concessions were necessary.

Ride With Pride

No special concessions were made with another physical activity: horse riding.

Every time I heard something was good for kids with autism, Jon was there. When I noticed Jon had an affinity for horses, I mentioned to Larry and Jon about "equine therapy." Jon was eager to volunteer with the Ride With Pride Program. Jon and I thought it would be a great experience for him. He could learn about caring for the horses, be trained to help children with disabilities, have a great day at the ranch, and be able to ride when he was there.

From the beginning Jon did not tell the owners of the ranch he was autistic. Therefore, they worked him pretty hard mucking stalls, bathing horses, cleaning hooves, and cleaning water bowls. It was very hot in the valley and sometimes I worried about heat stroke. Even though Jon never got the opportunity to ride, he worked tirelessly for the cause, gave many weeks of his time to the organization. That's the kind of person Jon is, a man of honor.

CHAPTER 10

Jon's Team

I assembled my own team around Jon: Mrs. Hurley, Hattie Brown, Master Lee, and tutors Arlene Fajnor, Phyllis Malone, and Brian Hoyt. Our housekeeper Gilda became a trusted family member. She knew how to bring out the best in Jon. She would play with him as a peer. There were many happy moments between some of the madness.

Belatedly, when Jon was older, we learned about Dr. Ivar Lovaas, a Norwegian-American clinical psychologist at UCLA, who advocated strict behavior modification for children with autism, starting before age 3½.

Lovaas would say, "We don't cure autism . . .That would mean we remove the neurological deviation. We help them obtain a normal life."

So convinced was Lovaas that applied behavior analysis was effective in childhood interventions, he said, "If I got Hitler here at UCLA at age 4 or 5, I could have raised him to be a nice person." (See Chapter 26 for more information on Lovaas.)

Why the Lovaas method works for some children and not others is not known. Lovaas would say in interviews, "There is no magic bullet," with which I wholeheartedly agree. Jon did not get treated in any way until age 5 ½. We didn't know much about Lovaas at the time, so we missed out on our chance to have him become part of our team and try his methods.

But God has made us like snowflakes. No two are alike. Therefore, not every method touted, as a miracle will give the results you crave. Some may even cause more chaos for you and your child. I'm glad, in a way, I never started Jon on the Lovaas method. I believe it would have been too disruptive and stressful for our family. Even tried-and-true methods often created more stress for Jon. For example, one tool most parents rely on for extinguishing inappropriate behavior is the "time out." When Jon was particularly difficult to manage, we would employ this method, but instead of getting Jon to calm down, his unruly behavior would escalate to the point of no return. His shrieking and banging in the other room was unrelenting and horrifying. We gave up on time outs and found that leaving the room or holding him firmly (the holding method) worked for our son. Seek and you will find. Never give up hope for your child's happy future. Do not continue employing methods that don't fit for you and your child. Many new advances in medications and treatments exist. Some will be almost like a miracle in your lives.

SECTION II

MIDDLE YEARS

CHAPTER 11

Managing Middle School

The difficulty in finding the right middle school was one of my most challenging endeavors. I am a psychotherapist by trade for a reason. I like being a peacemaker. Having to fight with the Los Angeles Unified School District was the last thing I wanted. The struggle to persuade them to do the right thing for Jon was so intense that I started drinking. I never drank in college or early adulthood. The pressure of raising a child with autism and constantly fighting for his rights was so hard for me to handle. Let me clarify "drinking": one or two drinks a day and no more. Even though the relaxation they brought was fabulous, I knew I had to be careful to take care of myself for Jon.

The main problem I encountered when placing Jon in middle school was his uniqueness. I admit I overprotected Jon. Wilbur Elementary School had been a small, nonthreatening environment. Even so, there I enlisted Miss Hattie Brown to look after him.

So, I knew Parkman Middle School was not a good fit. The middle school for Woodland Hills did not have a good reputation. A number of tough kids attended, bussed in from the inner city where fighting was the way they had learned to survive. But that was not the problem. The real problem was getting Jon into the right school for him.

Jon was now mainstreaming and fitting in with his peers, but I knew he was still sensitive and a bit naïve. Street-smart middle schoolers could chew him up and spit him out for lunch. The ratio of 30 or more students to a single teacher would be too distracting for Jon's focusing problems. Also, the teacher would not have the extra time to repeat things if Jon's processing issues required it.

The school district recommended special ed classes for autistic children and gave my husband and me a list of classes offered. They suggested we find the right ones for Jon.

I knew in my heart Jon did not need to go back to special ed, but I went through the motions. I patiently sat through several placements and promptly crossed them off the list. As I had suspected, Jon was much higher functioning at this point to thrive in those classes. We had worked so hard to get him to this point. I did not want Jon to backslide or to pick up inappropriate behaviors. I wanted a school that challenged him intellectually and was a good fit socially. Socially, Jon had very good self-esteem. I always told him how special I thought he was and praised him for his dancing and martial arts talents.

So, when I reported back to the school district that I found their suggestions unsatisfactory, I got the cold shoulder.

"Mrs. Wallace, if you can't find any of our district classes acceptable, then you are on your own," I was told. "If you find something that meets your needs, let us know. Maybe the district will fund that school, if we find it appropriate for Jon."

Thus began an exhaustive search for the best school I could find. When I found Westmark School, I thought I had died and gone to heaven! The Westmark campus looked more like a posh summer camp than an institution, with a little red schoolhouse library and classrooms around a swimming pool. The vibe was friendly and upbeat. No fear of violence or drugs on this campus. Visitors had to pass inspection by the friendly, but firm, security guard. No one was allowed on campus without a decal on the car window or visitors pass from administration. The teacher-to-student ratio was 12 students to one teacher—perfect for Jon. I was over the moon about the school! Plus, Westmark catered to learning differences such as dyslexia and processing problems.

I entered the administration office with a spring in my step to meet with Betsey Breese, the admissions staffer. Betsey was so friendly and welcoming; I liked her immediately. We spoke for a long time about my dilemma over Jon's placement. She understood the problem I had been facing. But although we had a nice meeting, Betsey said she could not admit Jon. Westmark did not have any autistic children because they were not equipped to meet that challenge. She felt it might be beyond their scope of expertise in teaching Jon, so admitting him would not be a good fit. I left heavy hearted with only one school to check out.

Bridges Academy

With my back against the wall, I entered the school. The principal was kind and explained how special her school was. I could not see that from the school campus—a bit too small and dreary. All the children at Bridges were doing work two years above their grade level, the principal said, and the teacher-to-student ratio was 3 to 1. I thought that was almost private instruction. I was sure Jon would excel academically but was not sure he would have the environment to flourish socially. But I couldn't see an alternative at the time, so we enrolled Jon at Bridges.

Jon's teachers were capable and willing participants in his education. Math was becoming less of a problem for Jon and he was working at advanced levels. A school requirement was foreign language lessons, in Japanese! At the end of that year I assessed his progress. His academic instruction was very good, but his social needs were unmet, almost as if he was being home schooled. I hadn't chosen that route because I knew my son needed stimulation from peer interaction.

Also, Bridges lacked a physical education program. Jon's recreation amounted to sliding down the cement walls of the Sepulveda Dam reservoir. He would come home threadbare daily. He was so thin compared to his height that all of his clothes were custom made, making his recreation quite costly. Besides, this was not my idea of P.E. I knew Jon was in desperate need of more socialization and physical education like soccer, basketball, swimming, or other activities. Theater training like that offered at Westmark would be fantastic.

So, I set up another meeting with Betsey Breese at Westmark. This time, I armed myself with charts, statistics, and laws, including the Chanda Smith consent decree that required the school district to educate special education students consistent with state and federal special education and civil rights laws.

I was prepared to fight for Jon's right to go to Westmark. Betsey could see my determination and probably knew I wouldn't go quietly. After some begging on my part, she gave in, saying, "It was good timing coming at the end of the school year. By doing so, summer school is about to begin. This way, Jon can go to summer school at Westmark. At the end of summer session, a committee will evaluate Jon's progress and adjustment to the school and let you know if he would be able to attend in the fall."

I was so happy. I knew this was the school for us and I had no fears about Jon doing well.

The summer flew by and we were told the good news: Jon was accepted into the 7th grade at Westmark School. Best news was the Los Angeles School District admitted that Westmark was the best fit for Jon. Because they lacked alternatives to suit his particular needs, they decided to fund his education. This was a fantastic outcome after all the blood, sweat, and tears I put into this endeavor. It was like winning the lottery! We were blessed and I thank God daily for this incredible outcome. Getting into Westmark meant overcoming a great hurdle, but I was not deluded into complacency. Jon's entrance into school did not end my nerve-wrenching daily search, seize, and rescue missions. Every day I would search for new information that might help our son. I would seize all the new information about autism regarding advances in medicine, treatments, and therapies. I would "rescue" him with tutoring, pet therapy, swimming with the dolphins, hypnotherapy, and medication trials.

CHAPTER 12

Endless Tasks and Professional Opinions

Endless second, third, and even more tests and professional opinions are one of the hardest things to deal with, especially when others doubt the diagnosis, including family members. As Jon progressed, he did better and better. This led to comments like, "Are you sure he's autistic? It's hard to believe!" So much doubt in others would rub off on me, eventually. Maybe B.J. [Dr. Freeman] was wrong, but I highly doubted it. Nonetheless, I subjected Jon to needless testing and stress. Test results from Dr. Martha Jura at UCLA and Dr. Andrew Wang, a psychiatrist, were bittersweet. I knew I was doing the right thing for my son; yet, I also knew that no matter how great Jon was doing he was still my autistic hero...I remembered the words of Dr. Lovaas. "Autistic children are not cured, that would be removal of the neurological deviation. We help them obtain a normal life."

Even though your child may be normalizing to their life circumstances, be aware they still face mighty challenges. Imagine coping with the stress of our times with autism; most of us can barely handle that. They will have to persevere with the "typicals," yet burdened by hypersensitivity to sound and labile emotionality, as well as processing problems, speech delays, hyperactivity, sleepless nights, allergy, and digestive disorders, and in some cases intellectual delays.

Think of your children as the superheroes of our time. They will always have to try harder and overcome so many obstacles just to live daily.

That's why I have one big pet peeve. Sometimes a person will look at your child and say they are getting privileges that the "typicals" aren't getting. Especially, when homework assignments are modified and test times are stretched to accommodate your child's processing problems. I could scream!

And never let any teacher or teacher's aide convince you that asking for things for your child is not fair to other children. That's the biggest crock I've ever heard. Don't even dignify that statement with an answer.

CHAPTER 13

Chelation Therapy and Vaccine Poisoning

As I researched chelation therapy for my fibromyalgia, I became aware of research indicating chelation as a therapy for children with autism. Mercury from many vaccines was suspected as the cause of some cases of autism. Remove the mercury and improve the condition. As the mother of a special needs child, I was willing to try just about anything to help my son.

Since that time, controversy has arisen surrounding chelation therapy for children with autism. Some deaths have occurred from heavy doses of chelating agents given intravenously.

Chelation therapy involves administering chelating agents to remove heavy metals from the body. The most common forms of heavy metal toxicity involve lead, arsenic, and mercury. Ethylene Diamine Tetra Acetate (EDTA) is used intravenously and is the treatment of choice for lead poisoning. Other chelating agents such as 2 3-dimercapto-1-propanesulfonic acid (DMPS) and alpha lipoic acid (ALA) are also used in conventional alternative medicine.

Based on the now-discredited hypothesis that mercury poisoning may trigger the symptoms of autism, chelation therapy is widely used by alternative therapists to treat autism. Some surveys suggest 2 to 8% of children with autism have undergone the therapy. Parents have a doctor provide treatment for lead poisoning or buy unregulated supplements. We fell into the ranks of those buying unregulated supplements. At the time, we were trying everything we could to help Jon. We understood that healing took place in increments and no one thing was the magic bullet. Nutritional supplements seemed a safe way to go. Removing excess mercury made sense to us at the time.

Jon and I went through four to six weeks of therapy, consisting of ingesting a chelating agent to pull mercury from the body to be excreted in the urine. The rub is the method also pulls and excretes many essential vitamins and minerals from the body, as well. So much so, that sometimes the patient can be left worse off.

Today, Aspies for Freedom, an autistic rights organization, considers use of chelation therapy unethical and potentially dangerous. Strong epidemiological evidence exists that refutes links between environmental triggers, in particular thimerosal-containing vaccines and the onset of autistic symptoms. In short, no scientific support for chelation therapy to treat autism exists.

Indeed, chelation therapy can be hazardous when used inappropriately. In August 2005, chelation therapy conducted by a member of ACAM, the American College for Advancement in Medicine, killed a 5-year-old boy with autism. A 3-year-old non-autistic girl died in February 2005, and a non-autistic adult died in August 2003. These deaths were due to cardiac arrest during chelation therapy caused by hypocalcemia, or low levels of calcium in the blood. EDTA should not be used to treat children. More than 30 deaths have been recorded in association with IV-administered disodium EDTA since the 1970s.

At the time we tried chelation for Jon, none of the above-mentioned deaths had taken place. Our quest for knowledge started 20 years ago. This was just the beginning of the new epidemic in autism. A lot of therapies were just starting to be used for "off label" purposes. Since then, so many more studies and research have been done. But I am always cautious with new treatments; therefore, Jon was given nutritional supplements. He did not have IV treatment and his therapy consisted of one round of treatment.

We did not repeat the therapy after the first time. I felt that if he had high amounts of mercury, the toxic levels had probably been reduced. That was good enough for me. I did not feel any different after treatment. Jon seemed to be a little calmer and he focused slightly better.

Our use of chelation therapy brings me to a major point I would like to make. Guilt of any kind can stop you in your tracks. Your life will not flow properly; your health and happiness will suffer. I could have felt guilty about failing to provide Jon early treatment at two years of age instead of waiting until he was 5 ½ years old. And I did feel guilty . . . for about 5 minutes. Reading the new findings later about chelation therapy, I could have cowered in a corner with shame. I didn't!

Later on, I will tell you one more mistake I made along the way for which I could have beaten myself bloody but didn't. The reason I gave myself a pass on all of these, was because of the incredible love and good intentions I had when I made decisions for my son. That's why I say: Always do what's in the best interest of your child. Will you make a few mistakes? You're damn right you will! No one is perfect. Perfection belongs in heaven. So, don't waste a minute of your precious time lamenting about spilt milk. Get on with the business of making a great life for yourself and your family.

In all matters, it's best to start slowly and proceed with caution under a doctor's care. The long, hard road of trial and error can take its toll on a family. But, this is something we will have to endure on our journey to recover our children.

That brings me back to the subject of snowflakes. Just because the latest research says that chelation therapy does not appear to be effective with autistic children, doesn't mean it hasn't helped anyone, anywhere. We all respond differently to foods, medications, and interventions.

Think about how many moms make their youngsters peanut butter and jelly sandwiches for school lunches—thousands. One peanut butter and jelly sandwich can kill my son, Jon, and my friend Marlene's son, Jeffrey.

Cancer treatments work so well for some, while other patients die. Some patients die from the treatments themselves.

When it comes to the vaccine controversy and thimerosal poisoning from vaccines, do I think it causes autism? Yes and no. In the majority of cases, the answer is no. In some cases I think it's yes!

I can remember one instance that stands out in my mind. I mentioned earlier one precious person that helped us raise Jon, Gilda, our housekeeper and companion to Jon. She had the patience of a saint while handling some nasty moods and meltdowns not for the faint of heart. Gilda stayed with us seven years until just a couple of weeks before she delivered her son, Albert. By then, she was family to us and I was quickly asked to be a godmother to Albert. Albert was such a beautiful boy with the largest brown eyes and beautiful eyelashes I had ever seen. His eyes were a wonder to behold.

One day, when my husband Larry and I were visiting Gilda's house, she said Albert was not feeling well. He was running a high fever from the vaccinations he had just received. The moment I saw the baby, I knew something was wrong. The light in his eyes had gone out and was replaced by a blank stare. I whispered to Larry, "Do you see what I see?"

We left a little later with questions on our minds. Not more than six months later, Albert was diagnosed with autism. How ironic. Gilda had spent seven years helping us raise our boy with autism; now she would face the same challenges. She had learned a thing or two from me and that was good. Albert began special classes by age 2.

We were now part of the larger family, the family of parents raising children with autism.

CHAPTER 14

The Power of Prayer

Can Prayer Heal People? I believe it does. My pastor, Joel Osteen, often tells a story about his mother, Dodie Osteen.

"My mother was sent home to die with terminal cancer, that was 30 years ago," he said. "It seems my mother refused to believe it was her time, so she affirmed and prayed to God every day. She thanked the Lord for healing her and spoke words of faith upon her life. 'Dear Lord, I am grateful that every day I'm getting stronger and becoming healthier.' Even when she felt awful and everything seemed contrary to her prayers, she continued and God rewarded her faith with a full recovery!"

As science investigates connections between mind and body, some scientists have found a person's faith can help him or her live a longer, healthier life. Just as meditation has been proven to improve health and quality of life, prayer has the same ability to relax a person in a state of high anxiety. By reducing stress, many health benefits abound. Lowering blood pressure and the heart rate, for example, are important factors in improving the immune system.

In my experience, I believe strongly that God had something mighty powerful to do with Jon's recovery. Every day for three years I would get on the treadmill and dedicate my workout to Him. As I would run I would repeat the mantra, "Dear Lord, today I dedicate this workout to you. I don't ask for anything for myself. I will face my health issues bravely. I will not ask for any divine intervention with my songs or my books. Just grant me the most important favor, and that is, make Jonnie well!"

For three years it was the same place, same thing, same place. One day, I got on the ridiculous machine and began to chant the mantra. In a loud, clear, magnificent voice God spoke to me.

"You can stop now, he is fine."

So, I got off the treadmill and never ran on that thing again. About that time in our process, I could see great strides were being made by Jon. I began to believe light existed at the end of the tunnel.

CHAPTER 15

Dr. Mark DeAntonio and Medications

When Jon was a little boy, I tried desperately to keep him off meds, despite a short trial with Ritalin in kindergarten. I just felt that I didn't want to do anything that would interfere with my child's developing and growing brain. We all know medications might have side effects, but we also know that sometimes they are a godsend or lifesaving proposition.

Around age 13 Jonnie had come a long, long way. He was totally caught up with his peers academically. He didn't need tutors to do his homework any longer. He was finally growing at an appropriate rate. Everyone loved him socially, which was so gratifying to my husband and me.

The one major problem that still existed was "homecoming." When Jon walked through the door we never knew what to expect. The frustrations of the day would be released on us in anger and tantrums. Jon could not help himself. He would express extreme sadness over his behavior, always ending the episode with "I love you guys."

I wanted to have a happy home for all of us. Therefore I met with Dr. Mark DeAntonio at the NPI (Neuropsychiatric Institute) at UCLA to open a discussion about medication. Dr. DeAntonio is a highly regarded doctor who treats adolescents with autism.

From the beginning, I liked Dr. DeAntonio a lot. I could tell he wasn't guessing when he made suggestions; his observations and suggestions came with loads of experience. Dr. D. instilled me with confidence about the medication trial on which we were about to embark. When I say trial, I mean it. Remember the "snowflakes": every one of us so unique that meds must be individually tailored to your child's specific needs and brain chemistry.

Jon was given Lexapro as an antianxiety medication, not for depression. Thank God Jon has not had to deal with depression. His tantrums were controlled beautifully with Risperdal, 2 mg, a very low dose. Many adjustments were made in the dosage; we went up ½ mg and down ½ mg several times until we reached the "sweet spot." I really mean "sweet spot." Today, we are all happy, getting along just fine. It really is home sweet home. So, don't be discouraged if your child would benefit from medication. So many of us need to take our meds, too! And this is probably the one area of our lives that is made better through chemistry.

CHAPTER 16

Methylation Pathway Disruption and Glutathione

Five years ago I was very surprised when I was diagnosed with breast cancer. It came out of nowhere. No one in my family tree ever had breast cancer. My 90-year-old mother was healthy and still had her two breasts! I did not have a harmful, mutated BRACA gene, which increases cancer risk.

I was obsessed with figuring out why this happened. Thus, began an exhaustive search for causes of cancer other than genetics. I discovered the unbelievable amount of toxins we are all exposed to on a daily basis.

You may wonder, What does this have to do with autism? A whole lot! Just bear with me a little longer.

My doctor at the time was Dr. Uzil Reiss who ran a panel of tests to ascertain if I had any genetic vulnerability to toxins in the environment. Oh my God! I couldn't believe what he found.

"It seems, young lady, you do not methylate properly," he told me. "Your ability to rid yourself of everyday toxins is compromised. Therefore, be careful with car exhaust, fireplace smoke, secondhand smoke, smoke from barbecues or any other sources."

I had a screwed-up methylation pathway. I immediately began eating organic foods to avoid pesticides and began using safe cosmetics, soy candles, safe cleaning products, and other substances.

When I decided to write this book about autism, I hoped to help other parents by sharing our struggles and triumphs. I wanted to give the gifts of knowledge and hope to others. My biggest surprise came with researching other sources as references for this book. I hadn't figured out the link between my own health and Jon's autism. As I read *Healing and Preventing Autism*, Dr. Jerry Kartzinel/McCarthy's book, I read about our autistic kids having methylation problems. Why hadn't I made that connection? Of course, Jon would have methylation problems like his mom; in my case it caused cancer, in Jon's case autism! I had already used the no VOC (volatile organic compounds) paint in his bathroom, gotten rid of pressed board furniture, and fed him organic food, if possible. I did not know about the protocol for this problem. I was amazed at the steps that can be taken to rectify the situation. By seeking to help others, Jon and I were given a great gift. I took him to his internist, Dr. Shafipour, the next week to discuss the regimen that would help both of us live better lives.

Glutathione

Glutathione is major antioxidant produced by the body. Without a robust methylation pathway, glutathione will not be produced properly. Without enough glutathione our immune system cannot do its job, which is to detoxify our bodies. Because Jonnie and I are low in glutathione we cannot detox the mercury in our flu shots, pesticides in our food, toxins in the environment, and toxic substances in our medications.

Protocol for raising glutathione

To raise glutathione levels, B_{12} shots are recommended. Off and on, I had been giving myself these shots, even though some of my doctors thought it had merely a placebo effect. I was sure it wasn't. Sometimes I was so tired I hardly had the energy to breathe, but after a B_{12} shot I would feel normal for two to three weeks.

Glutathione can be administered intravenously, by patch, or by using a nebulizer. I have also been taking folic acid and N-Acetyl Cysteine to aid the methylation pathway. Combined with doses of TMG (Trimethylglycine), you are likely to increase your total glutathione levels.

CHAPTER 17

Too Good to be True

If something is too good to be true, it usually is! We all know this adage, but when it comes to our own lives we are often too busy to pay attention. This happened to me a few times in my life and I hope I have learned my lesson, now. When it comes to friends for your children, especially as they grow older and a bit more independent, you need to beware, as this story illustrates!

One day Jon came home in total excitement. "I met someone on the beach."

"Oh, who is it?" I asked.

"I met the most interesting man," he enthused.

"Tell me about this guy," I said.

We live very close to Venice Beach, which attracts a lot of strange characters. I hung on every word as Jon explained that a young man was doing martial arts on the boardwalk. So, Jon, with his knowledge of martial arts, joined in. Soon, several people had gathered to watch. Jon began demonstrating some of his martial arts moves, which attracted an older man who stood by Jon and then began executing his own form of martial arts. The older man and Jon found out they had much in common. Martial arts and cooking (I had enrolled Jon in a chef's course), but the most extraordinary thing was both desired to be monks. As a matter of fact, Ryan, as the man was named, had been a monk. He showed Jon photos of himself dressed in monk's attire at a monastery.

"This all sounds very interesting Jon," I told my excited son. "But I'm not going to let you hang out with someone old enough to be your father unless I meet him first."

At the time, Jon was heavily into Hinduism and actively searching for a guru. A guru is someone who has studied a tradition you are interested in and has attained advanced status or enlightenment. The more the two conversed, the more Jon began to believe this person could be his teacher. Ryan encouraged this in Jon and even let him call him "teacher" instead of using his name.

Soon, Ryan was invited to our home. He came bearing gifts and insisted on cooking a meal for us. He said Jon was spiritually advanced (something I already knew). Ryan said he would be honored to lead Jon on his way to fulfilling his dreams.

I couldn't believe this distinguished man in a business suit was cooking for us and wanting to teach Jon spiritual lessons for absolutely no compensation. I didn't know exactly what to make of this, but God does sometimes work in mysterious ways.

"When the student is ready, the teacher will appear," right? I took Ryan's business card and checked out his employment. He was indeed employed as an office manager.

I reasoned with myself, "This guy has a job; he didn't look as if he drinks, smokes, or takes drugs. He is celibate because he is still a practicing monk. He genuinely seems to like Jon and Jon usually gets along much better with adults than people his own age. OK!"

I would permit this friendship, with a watchful eye.

As the weeks went by the two of them became very close. Ryan would spend endless hours reading religious books to Jon and taking him on all kinds of excursions. They went to numerous temples, spiritual sites, and Chinese herbalists, plus cooked together. Ryan was a massage therapist and gave Jon lengthy massages to open his chakras. Ryan became part of our family.

Not too long afterward, a very close friend of mine invited me to her beautiful cabin in Lake Arrowhead for a weekend with a couple of friends to celebrate my birthday. I invited Ryan and Jon and my friend, Mary. I knew the beautiful view of the pines and lake would be highly appreciated by Ryan and Jon. They could meditate and read in a very peaceful place.

The cabin consisted of three bedrooms and two bathrooms. My friend Sonnie and I shared the beautiful master bedroom on the upper floor. Jon and Ryan bunked together. They shared a bathroom with my good friend Mary. Sonnie and I couldn't believe what fun we were having. Ryan cooked for us. He took pictures of all of us the entire weekend. We saw Jon and Ryan studying spiritual books on the deck and meditating to their hearts' content.

I felt very blessed to have such good friends. It made my birthday so special.

All good things sometimes have to come to an end, so they say.

When we returned home, I noticed Jon was behaving strangely. He said things like, "Ryan can control the traffic with his mind. He just walks into chaos in the road and all the cars go into slow motion and part to let us pass."

There were other psychotic statements regarding Ryan's powers.

Soon after this kind of talk, Jon became very ill. I discovered that Ryan had talked Jon into fasting to emaciation and stopping all medications cold turkey. This kind of thing can kill a person.

"You are the reincarnation of St. Francis," Ryan had told Jon. "God will help you overcome the detox."

Jon and I were so close and we discussed everything together. Now, this other person was making extremely important decisions for my son. And Jon was confiding in him.

Jon and I sat together hugging for a long time. We discussed the dangers of what Ryan had done. Then the bombshell came down. Ryan had a method to his madness. He would get Jon into a state to be compromised mentally and then propose outlandish ideas to him. Jon felt so betrayed.

Parents often will do anything for children, including taking unusual requests into consideration. Remember, Jon had some difficulty connecting to his peers, many of whom were into drinking and smoking and sex. Jon was into spirituality big time. Therefore, I let him engage in this unusual friendship. I wanted him to have a close friend.

Now, I realize Jon needs to be more selective and choose friends his own age with common interests, even if that means a little loneliness sometimes.

CHAPTER 18

Jon's Team Becomes a Village

By Jon's middle years, I had learned how critical the right school placement is for a child. I had trusted my instincts as a parent and not permitted others to talk me out of my feelings. And I had reached out to others and to treatments, even though sometimes, as I have shown, it wasn't always the right decision. But you will always need help. So, don't be afraid to reach out to others and build a village around your child for their best life and chance for success.

By his middle years, Jon's team had expanded to a village. Here are the people that he included:

Mom and Dad, love and support
Gilda Gijaro, loving companion and playmate to Jon
Dr. Mark DeAntonio, Psychiatrist
Dr. B.J. Freeman, NPI (Neuropsychiatric Institute), UCLA
Dr. Jondron, Children's Hospital for growth hormone
Dr. Garb, asthma and allergy
Master Lee, physical education Tae Kwon Do
Dr. Robert Smith, Pediatric dentist
Dr. Sharon Crowder, Orthodontic dentist
Dr. Bud Zukow, Pediatrician
Dr. McLaren, Pediatrician
Dr. Solomon, family doctor
Dr. Shafipour, internist
Arlene Faynor, tutor
Phyllis Malone, tutor
Brian Hoyt, IABA (Institute for Applied Behavior Analysis) resource person
Gary Lynn Wollard, dance
Dawn Kinkaide, dance
Nisha Fokes, dance
The State Street Ballet, Santa Barbara
Kate Fitzgerald, librarian at Westmark
Jean Smart, acting coach

Leslie Barnaby, Principal at Westmark
Betsey Breese, Administration at Westmark

The teachers at Westmark who went over and above the call of duty: Marcelo Frutos, football Coach Fox, Mr. Gruytch, Mr. Butterfield, Steve Haskal, and Charles Wingate

Alice Soto, Westside Regional Center
Debra Ansley Allen, respite provider
Sister Danielle Plancich and husband Jeff Plancich
Krista Laura and husband, Eric Laura
Marina Tae Kwon Do: Master Jones, Mrs. Jones, Mr. Lopez, Miss "B"
David Dorian Ross, Tai Chi master and mentor
Fari and Sue, Marina City Club Fitness
Stephen Orenstein, Brain Enhancement Institute
Todd Gewant, Chiropractor

Mom's best friends that she would leave me in an emergency without reservations: Sonnie and Lou Bergener, Donna Ollins, Pauline Crane, Marlene Tang, Elyn Avtal, Ansley Allen, Vee MacDonald, Mary and Tom Espinosa, and Nina Purtell.
Maryam Sarnot, Reconnective healing
Zhou Ting-Jue, Qi Gong master
The monks and teachings of Paramahansa Yogananda at the Lake Shrine
Dr. Klapper, renowned doctor of sports injury

If I have forgotten anyone, and I'm sure I have, please forgive me. I am sincerely sorry.

SECTION III

PRESENT

CHAPTER 19

Insights to Mothers on Raising an Autistic Child

In 2011, I attended an autism conference where Ricki Robinson, M.D., M.P.H, a clinical professor of pediatrics at USC Keck School of Medicine, was a guest speaker. Dr. Robinson began with the most important aspect of raising your special needs child, that is, the happy and fulfilled child. I always say the goal is to be happy; that's everything. Your child will need lots of support. I'm sure most of you parents are actively engaged in this right now.

Be aware that worry takes the place of action and can keep you stuck and unproductive. It's important to see opportunities that lie ahead. My dad used to follow the familiar expression and see the glass half full, instead of half empty. Your child's self-esteem is of the utmost importance to all parents. Can you go overboard? Sometimes. From the day I first laid my eyes on my son, Jon, I thought, "This is the most beautiful boy I have ever seen."

It has not changed much since then. He's my hero, overcoming so many challenges along the way. I tell him every day how much I love him, how smart and talented he is, and that he makes my life worth living.

Suffice it to say, Jonnie has fabulous self-esteem, and I know he's not going to take any guff from anyone. It makes me feel a little more assured about his quality of life after I'm gone. To maintain that self-esteem, never speak in the third person around your child. And remember children with autism have very keen hearing; they can hear through walls, therefore, be very careful what you say and where you say it!

Becoming Self-Sufficient

Begin early with responsibilities, such as chores. Most important of all, set limits. For the first three years of Jon's life, I admit I let him have his way but I didn't know he had autism. He was restless, demanding, and engaged in tantrums. I was determined to let him be a baby because I was slapped into submission from the moment I opened my eyes. When Jon spit out his food, I laughed and tried again. I did not set any limits because I wanted to wait until I was sure he could understand the process. I estimate we started around 4 years old. This was the time when Jonnie could finally go out in public and was expected to "behave" in pre-school. Because Jon was very verbal and smart, he adapted to following rules. Once I knew he could be socially appropriate, I didn't give him the chance to regress into inappropriate behaviors. From that time on, I always have stressed "please," "thank you," and sharing. I consider limit setting one of the most important concepts for you and your child. It could make the difference between a person who is well liked and fits in with others or one who doesn't. I consider building self-esteem and limit setting the cornerstone of raising any child successfully.

Teen Years

Do not make autism an excuse for unacceptable behavior. The teenage years are a minefield for parents of all children. Your teen wants to be his/her own person and that is normal. The tendency to see parents as "stupid" at this stage is part of the process of your child breaking free of your influence. Raging hormones and input from peers can exacerbate this problem.

What Can Be Done?

When I talk to my friends with "typicals," I remind them we hold the purse strings. Withholding money our teens want for the extra things "they can't live without," provides a powerful incentive for them to follow rules and be polite.

Contracts on which both parent and child agree are helpful when tensions arrive. Behavior therapy is useful with every teen. Reward the behaviors you want to encourage and extinguish the unwanted behaviors. You can extinguish unwanted behaviors by withholding spending money, outside activities, or just completely ignoring the negative "acting out."

The Walking Away Method

Whatever you do, it won't be easy, but as parent of children with autism, we have become warriors by the time they reach their teen years. Dr. Robinson says let go, but provide a soft landing! Allow your child to make mistakes. I'm still struggling with this one! Don't abruptly pull out resources and support.

With all that being said, our nonverbal children and children with severe sensory processing problems may appear to be misbehaving when, in fact, they are engaged in compensatory behaviors that calm their anxiety.

Dr. Barry Prizant gave a few examples of such behaviors:

#1 A child bolts out of the classroom. (Why? Because of severe anxiety.)

#2 Another child when presented with math homework, throws tantrums and won't comply. (Why? Because the work needs modification; it's just too difficult for this child.)

#3 A child aggressively pushes you out of his way to get where he is going. (Why? If children perceive danger, they will do anything necessary to get away.)

All these children appear to be misbehaving, when in actuality, they are surviving the best way they know how.

Also stimming (self-stimulating) and repetitive behaviors such as hand flapping and rocking are often perceived as "bad behaviors." But, these actions help the child self-regulate his moods and reduce anxiety. Therefore, I believe the child should be able to engage in self-soothing behaviors when necessary. Punishing a child who is already suffering does not make any sense and is downright cruel.

EXPLOSIVE TANTRUMS, AGGRESSION AND SELF-INJURIOUS BEHAVIOR (SIB)

Tantrums, aggression & SIB are some of the most upsetting scenarios that a child or family has to deal with. I only had to see Jon biting his arm one time, to tell you that it is a heart-breaking scene. With that being said, it is very important to understand neurotransmitter dysfunction. Neurotransmitter dysfunction is at the root of these behaviors. When the family understands the cause of the problem, effective treatment can be implemented to improve the situation.

Aggression can be the result of too much dopamine, which plays a role in impulse control. "If your child has an over active sensory profile, he can have an aggressive out burst triggered by increased anxiety, which might come from a decreased understanding of environmental and emotional cues." Rickie Robinson, M.D.

Low serotonin can cause anxiety and aggressive out burst. Selective serotonin reuptake inhibitors (SSRIs) are effective for this condition.

"Post-episode remorse is enormous and the outbursts may remain upsetting to him so for some time. Soothing your child using techniques that you know work and not adding "fuel to the fire" by either shouting or disciplining him will help ease the situation." Ricki Robinson, M.D.

When increased dopamine is suspected for aggressive behavior, the neuroleptics Risperdal and Abilify have been FDA approved for this treatment. In Jon's case low dose Risperdal coupled with an SSRI for anxiety has eased the situation and made all of our lives more peaceful and happy.

Another very important aspect is allowing your child to say no! This is an important tool to help your youngster to feel empowered. And always ask why, when your child says no. You will uncover the struggles they are going through and their reasons for not wanting to do something.

You will be surprised at the insights you will gain into your child's quirky behaviors, allowing both of you to live together compatibly and compassionately.

Life enrichment experiences, religion, and spirituality have always been important to Jon and are a major focus in his life. They bring him great pleasure and make him the wonderful person he is today.

Vacations

Jon is always happy on our family vacations. I believe they give him respite from always thinking about his future. On vacations, we all live in the moment—so nice! He loves visiting relatives in Italy, learning the Italian language, and experiencing European culture.

If trips to Europe are not in your budget, a change of scenery, such as camping or flying or driving to visit relatives in a different town or state, or even just setting aside a few days at home to explore local sites, can provide the same benefits.

Interests

Jon is vigorously pursuing his individual talents and interests. Among these interests are martial arts, dance, and community service.

April is autism awareness month. Recently, Jon and I made a commitment to raise money for the cause. We have agreed to work hard at this venture and have an event every April as long as we are able to do it. Last week, unbeknownst to me, Jon and his friends made over 100 sandwiches, put them in paper bags with inspirational messages, and delivered them to the homeless population in Venice Beach. Way to go Jon and company!

Individuals with autism can have rich, productive lives. Be hopeful your child will find the right path for his or her life.

For my son, Jon, his interest in martial arts has blossomed into a career. He will pursue a fitness professional credential. He recently became credentialed as a Tai Chi instructor and will seek additional skills as a teacher of martial arts for the general population and for those with special needs.

"Don't allow ceilings. There are not time limits! Learning is lifelong." R. Robinson, author of *Autism Solutions.*

CHAPTER 20

What Martial Arts Has Meant to Me by: Jon Wallace

I love martial arts with all my heart. It is a beautiful expression of life. That is when it's used in the right way. I don't agree with the fighting organizations such as the UFC (Ultimate Fighting Championship), where people beat each other to a bloody pulp. The only time a person can justify physically hurting another human being is in defense of self or others. Not as a form of brutal entertainment. Let's not regress back to the day of gladiator fights in Rome.

Martial arts, as a form of defense, makes sense to me. I am able to walk around and feel confident in my ability to be safe. This does not mean if you learn martial arts that you're automatically free from the possibility of harm; therefore, we are always taught to avoid confrontation whenever possible. The best defense is walking away when you can.

Martial arts has allowed me to carry myself with confidence and comfort; what a beautiful thing!

Another fantastic benefit of martial arts is that it is a great form of exercise; and exercise is awesome for everyone.

You don't have to be an exceptional athlete to practice martial arts. Just because you can't do the splits all the way down or kick your feet above your head, doesn't mean you can't enjoy your practice and reap lots of benefits.

I love martial arts exercise. It has done incredible things for me. It keeps my mind and body in great shape. Often after exercising in martial arts class, I feel very energetic, happy, peaceful, clear-minded, and, overall, fantastic. I believe with all my heart that exercise through the martial arts can do magnificent things for autistic people, as it has done for me. Remember, exercise enhances the mind and body, and also releases hormones, increases energy, and does other phenomenal things to give a person good health, VOILÀ!

Last, but not least, martial arts are a spectacular way to socialize and have team camaraderie. So many autistic kids feel lonely and isolated. In the dojo, they will feel a sense of belonging and happiness. Select your dojo carefully and be sure the vibe is friendly, welcoming, and resonates with you. That is what my dojo is like—very positive, uplifting, and near and dear to my heart. My dojo members are my extended family. They are my martial arts family. This new family will build up your self-confidence, make you feel accomplished, and a more happy you, golden!! So if you are intrigued by the idea of trying martial arts, I say go out there and give it a shot. That's enough rambling for now. Just do it!

Cheers! Jon Wallace

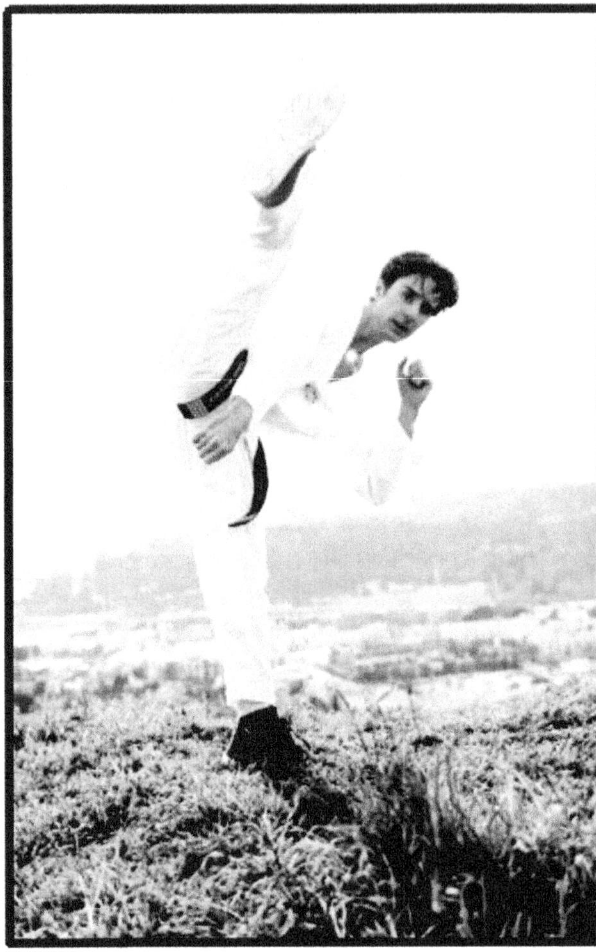

NO LONGER TINY BUT STILL MIGHTY

CHAPTER 21

Brain Enhancement Institute and Neuroplasticity

My husband, Larry, loves his cup of Joe in the morning with his friends. And I love that he has a morning ritual that brings him enjoyment.

One day he returned from coffee with a request that I meet his friend, Stephen, who has a center called BEI Institute in Playa del Rey. The center works with children and adults who struggle with issues related to neurodysfunction, including addictions and learning disabilities.

"I don't know, Larry," was my initial response. "That's another whole commitment. And how much is this going to cost?"

Then I thought, we have good health insurance. If this program is covered by our insurance, I would feel better about going ahead. I realized insurance companies would not cover something that was experimental or bogus.

We gave Stephen our insurance information, and he made us a deal we couldn't refuse: What was not covered by our insurance would be waived.

Jon started his program with brain maps and consultations. Larry and I always felt well-informed about our child's obstacles and progress.

Jon went to the Brain Enhancement Institute (BEI) three times a week for one year. He was happy to comply with treatment because the staff was very kind and Jon, himself, could see he was steadily improving. The brain training was like playing video games that challenged his thinking abilities not just hand-eye coordination.

After the year was complete Jon graduated the program with "flying colors." He had raised his IQ as promised by the center. He did not need to continue; he was told "just get on with life Jon, you are very capable."

I was impressed that the team did not encourage further treatment that may not have reaped any benefits. As promised we did not have to pay a balance, even though our insurance had stopped paying somewhere along the way. Thank you, Stephen Orenstein.

Since a tsunami of autism cases is predicted for the future, hopefully the increased awareness and research will lead to recovering all of our children.

One new, recent discovery is brain plasticity, meaning that the brain has the ability to change, grow, and remap with learning. When certain areas are damaged, other centers in the brain take over the job by growing new connections. (Previously, it was assumed that the brain lacked the ability to increase synapses and neural connections!) We have come a long way with this discovery. Brain training for certain brain injuries and brain deficiencies now seems obvious. We can all have hope to improve our abilities and that is a good thing.

Neuroplasticity describes how experiences create neural pathways in the brain and these pathways can change location based on experiences or recovery from brain injury. Long-lasting functional changes in the brain occur when we learn new things or memorize new information. These changes in neural connections = neuroplasticity. An enormous amount of research has revealed that the brain never stops changing and adjusting.

CHAPTER 22

Meditation and Neuroplasticity: Jon's Views

A number of studies have linked the practice of meditation to differences in the brain's cortical thickness or gray matter density. One of the most well-known studies was published by neuroscientist Sara Lazar at Harvard University in 2000. Richard Davidson, a neuroscientist at the University of Wisconsin, has also researched meditation and its effect on the brain, leading experiments in cooperation with the Dalai Lama. His studies suggest that long-term or short-term practice of meditation results in different levels of activity in brain regions associated with attention, anxiety, depression, fear, and anger, and also affects the body's ability to heal itself. These functional changes may be caused by changes in the physical structure of the brain.

I asked Jon about meditation and he said that when he was contemplating becoming a monk, he meditated diligently. Sometimes, he would become agitated because he could not stop his thoughts from invading his mental, meditative space. But with practice and understanding, he progressed. Jon realized that he could welcome the thoughts and then dismiss them, watching them drift by, in itself a form of meditation. Jon is now able to meditate during many parts of his day, using breathing meditation, walking meditation, washing dishes meditation, and other forms. It's a matter of being in the moment, being exquisitely present in all of life.

Two physical conditions prompt Jon into the meditative state: submersing himself in the ocean and feeling a breeze caress his body. I told him that water and the rustling breezes in the trees also do it for me.

Whatever takes you there, go there! The benefits of meditation have been documented for many years.

For children who are anxious and spinning out of control, meditation may be one valuable resource in dealing with the complex puzzle we call autism.

CHAPTER 23

Growing Up Autistic: Trevor Pacelli with Contributions by Jon Wallace

Trevor Pacelli, 20 years old as of this writing, was diagnosed at age 5 with autism spectrum disorder. The telltale sign was that he was slow to learn to speak. Despite his early difficulty using words, Trevor nonetheless wrote *Six Word Lessons on Growing up Autistic: 100 Lessons to Understand How Autistic People See Life* (www.growingupautistic.com).

One day I opened my Costco magazine and came across a very interesting article by Fran R. Schumer. Ms. Schumer had interviewed Trevor and endorsed his book saying, "The organization of the books [is] charming, wittily autistic." Trevor was diagnosed was autism at the same time my Jonnie was diagnosed. I wondered what they shared in common besides being on the spectrum. So I asked Jon questions that correlate to statements made by Trevor in his book. This is what we found:

Some children with autism said they felt much better when they were highly structured with academic activities. I agree; Jon is definitely more fully functioning when his time is structured and he does not have time to ruminate and obsess about things.

Trevor mentioned he likes to plan his entire day—what he is going to do and for how long. Jon agrees, planning his entire day gives him a feeling of purpose and calm, but he does not plan the exact times and durations of each activity. (Mom thinks maybe he should.)

They get A's or F's in their schoolwork. Trevor and Jon have this in common. They can have tremendous gifts in certain areas. For Jon it's science, writing, dance, martial arts, and foreign language. Math eludes him.

Trevor says autistic kids need time to be alone, to unwind and "smell the petunias."

"I enjoy the company of friends and family, just not as much as most people."

To which Jon observed, "I agree. Time alone is good to unwind, but I prefer time with friends and family to alone time. I enjoy friends and family a lot."

Trevor: "The idea is in my head perfectly, but forming it into words is difficult and takes time."

Jon: "Every once in awhile I have that problem of word finding that is appropriate to the situation, but not so often."

Trevor: "Insults may be taken too personally . . . I have very sensitive emotions that get hurt easily."

Jon: "When I was young I was more emotionally raw, but now not so much anymore. I'm much more at peace and can see the insults as bad behavior on the other person's part and let it roll off my shoulders."

Trevor: "They hold onto their grudges, looking back 10 years ago, I am still annoyed at someone for either hurting my feelings or simply being an annoying pest."

Jon: "I don't hold grudges. It's a waste of time."

(I have to get Jon to help me in this area. My childhood memories sometimes rear their ugly heads, but not so much anymore.)

Trevor had difficulty with guilt and observed that "Realizing my wrongs brings down my spirits tremendously throughout the day."

His mom Pattie says, "Clearly explain that what they did wasn't so bad compared to what other kids their age often do in the same situation."

Jon: "Sometimes I can get down on myself if I feel I hurt someone's feelings or said the wrong thing in a particular situation."

Memories

Trevor: "With some autistic people, such as me, their memories are so precise that they remember the little details on a situation that others do not."

Jon: "I don't think my memories are that different from anyone else's, in my opinion."

Trevor: "Touch, sound, sight, taste, or smell, a child with autism is sensitive to anything extreme."

Jon: "Not for me."

Jon listens to very loud music, which jars me, and goes outside in the blazing sun without sunglasses (something that makes me crazy) but does not faze him. He is also more resistant to pain than others.

Give Them Patience—Let Them Think

Trevor: "If something comes up suddenly for me, I don't know how to take it. If I am given about 15 minutes to mull it over and process the thought, I can be more reasonable about accepting the change."

Jon: "I do feel that way, too."

So, as you can see, some similarities exist between people on the autistic spectrum, but it is also evident that they all have their own personality, likes, and dislikes. They should be treated accordingly.

CHAPTER 24

My Life with High Functioning Autism by: Jon Wallace

At times I have not been sure if I really am autistic. I feel so independent. I have traits that a lot of autistic people don't have, such as having good eye contact, forming strong bonds with others, and being very social. More recently, when I look back on my life, I have said to myself, "O.K., it makes sense that some doctors have said I am autistic. I do have the OCD (obsessive compulsive disorder), processing problems, and some quirky behavior. It can be confusing; after all, I don't know what it's really like to be a "neurotypical!"

I am at a very good place in my life now. I remember how—in the past—I used to have intense emotional issues. I had times when I would feel livid anger for no reason at all. My mom calls that extreme anger with no precipitating event. That was a main reason my mom had me evaluated, to see what was disturbing me so much. When I was asked about what made me so angry, I would come up with some reason, but the reasons were nonsensical and were not reasons at all.

Now that I think about B.J. Freeman's diagnosis of my autism and the temper tantrums I used to have, I can see why she came to that conclusion. I know I am somewhat psychologically and emotionally different from my peers, but that's OK with me. And my mom loves my depth of emotion and warm heart very much. I don't drink and smoke or have promiscuous sex either. Mom and I are very proud of that, too.

I have struggled greatly for many years (birth to 21 years old), so it seems to me I am probably on the spectrum.

I am now 24 years old and have come out of most of the autistic haze. I am doing wonderfully even though I still have some challenges I deal with at this time. I still have some nervousness and OCD. My challenges now are minor in comparison to the way they were before. But then I have come to realize everyone has their own difficulties to deal with unless you are some kind of saint or enlightened master.

I credit so many people and things to my rise.

But God has to come first on my gratitude list. He/She has provided the wind beneath my wings, enabled me to soar like an eagle, and play amongst the clouds, which led to my happiness and victory.

Thankfully, now, my OCD has calmed down and I don't have bouts of rage any longer. I actually consider myself a very happy person and a very kind person. I still have some arguments with my parents but much less than before. Probably as much as "neurotypicals." I'm sure my parents enjoy me much more than they did in previous times and I enjoy them much more, too. I try to be kind to everyone I encounter: friends, colleagues, people on the street, and the homeless. With the exception of those that may look questionable, then I stay away, but carry a kindness and unconditional love in my heart for them too.

At this time my anger is so little, one percent of what it used to be; and I'm rarely depressed, maybe once in a blue moon. Even so I strive to be better every day. I wish I could achieve perfection and maybe someday I will. People that are united with God and His cosmic energy are people that have attained healthy, happy, complete lives. They are balanced spiritually, mentally, emotionally, and physically, yes! I also feel that life is everlasting and that our spirit doesn't live just one physical life on Earth. It is my hope that all of us will achieve cosmic consciousness.

God has been a major support for me in my life. In addition to that support has been the constant care I received from my parents. My mother and father have been with me through thick and thin. If I didn't get this dedication that I had from them I wouldn't be where I am today. Thank you Mom and Dad. I love you fantastically, incredibly. And thank you to the rest of my family. I love you dearly.

I have been so blessed to receive great love from many people along the way. I have felt the love and kindness from friends, teachers, colleagues, neighbors, and many others, including complete strangers. The wonderful, warm, kindness I get from others has really touched my heart. Thank you all for your generosity. You have lifted me up and I have grown like Jack's beanstalk. Thank you, thank you.

Socialization has been profound for me. Most of us are social beings, even many of autistic individuals. It has felt great to reach out to people and have them reach back. The kindness I project towards them is returned to me and the great conversations have brought healing, happiness, restoration, and improvements in my life.

Life experiences have caused me to grow greatly. As a person has to navigate the world and explore different people and cultures, it stretches our perspectives. It's like a medicine to the mind. We are molded and shaped into a person of higher elevation than we were before. World travel has done this for me. My last trip to Europe enabled me to bond with relatives in Italy. I enjoyed that immensely and will be studying Italian to enhance that experience. Priceless!

Exercise and good nutrition, so important to me, have lifted me to a higher state of being. Exercise in the right way and right dose, has always helped me from the time I was a child. It is important for my mental and physical well-being. Mentally, it balances my moods and, physically, it keeps me in great shape and healthy. Exercise combined with everything else I am doing has me doing super fantastic, better than ever before. Part of good nutrition is eliminating things that cause us distress or allergic reactions. Eliminating coffee has also been a miracle in my life. My brain is much more caffeine sensitive than most people. When I would have a cup in the morning, I would be up all night until 8 or 9 a.m. the next day. Since I am challenged with sleep problems, it is an added burden.

Presently, I am still working on my sleep scenario. I am getting to bed 1 a.m. or 3 a.m., not great, but tremendously better than before. I am experimenting with natural sleep aids such as valerian and melatonin. I will see a sleep specialist next week. I want to get to bed by 10 p.m. or, at latest, 1 a.m., each night. That's my goal and I know I'll achieve it.

I have recently had the ALCAT test to test for food allergy and sensitivities. My mom and I will be working on allergy related issues to hopefully turn the final corner in my recovery.

I am very excited with where I am now and where I am going. Do not be terribly disheartened with a diagnosis of autism. There is life after diagnosis. So, be brave like the lion. Thank you for coming along for the ride. It has been a pleasure.

SECTION IV

MY RESEARCH

Parents of autistic children do not be discouraged or depressed upon hearing the diagnosis. It is an opportunity for tremendous growth and knowledge about the body and the substances that affect it. This knowledge can benefit not only your child, but you as well!

The next section contains just some of my research; the parts that I think you might find the most useful. Please be aware that it is just a jumping-off point. New findings are occurring every day, which gives us all hope!

CHAPTER 25

Early Intervention and Dr. Ivar Lovaas

Dr. Ivar Lovaas (May 8, 1927–August 2, 2010) was a Norwegian-American clinical psychologist at UCLA. In his original studies in the late 1950s, Dr. Lovaas used aversives, unpleasant stimuli that induce changes in behavior through punishment, such as electroshock. He successfully treated approximately 50% of individuals engaging in instances of extreme self-injury whose life expectancy was reduced by secondary infection. Later studies have focused on extinction methods, in which attention is given only when individuals are not engaging in self-injury.

Dr. Lovaas was the first researcher to suggest that, for some children, autism is treatable. He believed that after rigorous training, some autistic children would be able to catch up to their peers and function in conventional classrooms. He did not see any benefit to psychotherapy with autistic children. Instead, Dr. Lovaas took a behavioral approach. He proposed that autism could be ameliorated through a rigorous one-on-one program of behavior modification. The "Lovaas method" emphasizes intensive repetition: The autistic child works 35 to 40 hours a week with a teacher or parent. Dr. Lovaas stressed early intervention, with children ideally starting therapy before age 3 ½.

His operating model was a system of rewards and punishments intended to reinforce appropriate behaviors and discourage inappropriate ones. The occasional slap administered early on to discourage shrieking, head banging, and self-mutilation gave way to positive reinforcements, like food, affection, and tickling to reward children.

In 1987, Dr. Lovaas published a study in *The Journal of Consulting and Clinical Psychology*. The study of autistic 2- and 3-year-olds began in 1970. Most of the children in the study functioned at a low level and spoke very little, if at all. Nineteen received intensive behavior modification 40 hours a week for several years. By the time they were age 7, nine children had gained 30 IQ points and could attend regular first grade classrooms.

Children in the control group who received only 10 hours of weekly therapy showed little intellectual or social change. In a 1993 follow-up, the children who had gained IQ points maintained all their gains. In 1995, Dr. Lovaas founded the Lovaas Institute, based in Los Angeles, which trains teachers in his method. Today, thousands of children throughout the United States and abroad are receiving Lovaas therapy.

It is uncertain why the Lovaas method works for some children and not others. Lovaas would say in interviews, "There is no magic bullet." I wholeheartedly agree.

CHAPTER 26

Leaky Gut Syndrome

Because I have always been very interested in nutrition and biology, I make it a practice to watch Dr. Oz anytime I have a spare moment. I tape all the episodes and watch the ones I feel might help our family. My husband and Jon used to laugh at my dedication to the TV show, but along the way I think he and Jon have become semi-converts.

Recently, the show that intrigued me the most was called, "The disease most doctors can't diagnose." It turned out to be "Leaky Gut Syndrome."

Dr. Oz explained how "a battle is going on in this country and most people and doctors don't know it exists! The battle is on inside."

When we eat something it should go from mouth to anus without causing havoc on the body, he explained. The problem begins when the lining of the gut wall becomes damaged and therefore more permeable. This allows toxins to pass into the bloodstream instead of being eliminated. Nutrients, toxins, and proteins get through the lining, causing havoc in the body. Proteins need to be broken down into amino acids before they hit the bloodstream. If partial proteins enter the bloodstream, the body reacts with an immune response. In this way, substances get into our bloodstreams that should not be there!

<u>Symptoms</u>

Joint pain	Food sensitivity
Eczema	Fatigue
Psoriasis	Bloating/gas
Allergies	Abdominal cramps
	Diarrhea

Dr. Oz described the damage to the gut as scissors cutting large holes in the intestinal wall where only very tiny holes should exist. These holes let harmful things pass through that shouldn't.

The Scissors

1. Food allergy or sensitivity
2. Antibiotics
3. Excessive use of NSAIDs (nonsteroidal anti-inflammatory drugs)
4. High sugar diet
5. Parasites

The Test

A simple test, called the intestinal permeability test, can determine if Leaky Gut Syndrome exists. A patient simply drinks a special liquid containing both small and large molecules of sugar, and, later, sends a urine sample to Genova Diagnostics in Georgia (www.gdx.net). The urine is analyzed to see if the large molecules go through the gut. If so, the person, even a child, would have the condition.

What to do about "Leaky Gut?"

The Protocol

Remove:	Gluten
	Dairy
	Refined sugar
	Alcohol
	Nightshades (tomatoes, potatoes, eggplant)
	NSAIDs
	Antacids
Replace:	Eat fermented vegetables, such as sauerkraut
	Oil of oregano and garlic as natural antifungals
Repair:	Colostrums (which promotes repair of intestinal cells)
	Omega-3s
	Flaxseeds, walnuts, salmon
	Glutamine powder (aids in repairing lining)

So many of our children are suffering in silence. It is definitely worthwhile to do this simple test to eliminate any doubts about this sneaky condition. Remember, most doctors don't know about Leaky Gut or don't believe it exists. This is one of those times you will have to stand your ground.

Now that we opened a large can of worms about "Leaky Gut" and elimination diet, I'm afraid we will have to get into this lengthy subject and how it relates to autism. Under protocols to follow, Dr. Oz's segment suggested removing certain foods.

Gluten and dairy, mainly and first on the list, are both naturally occurring proteins. Gluten is found in wheat, barley, rye, and other grains. Casein is found in dairy products such as milk, cheese, and yogurt.

Dr. Oz emphasized removing these foods to help relieve symptoms of joint pain, eczema, allergies, fatigue, bloating, and intestinal distress. Currently, many websites tout "miraculous cures" for autistic children from the GFCF (gluten-free/casein-free) elimination diet that reduces their autistic behaviors. In the 1970s, a link was first made between gluten and casein and autism. So far, however, this theory remains unproven. The main premise is that autistic children do not digest properly and undigested peptides pass through their intestinal membranes because of Leaky Gut. These peptides enter the blood stream and cause all kinds of havoc physically, including the neurobehavioral symptoms that we call autism.

CHAPTER 27

Academy of Pediatrics—Autism Spectrum Disorders: What Every Parent Needs to Know

Leaky Gut Syndrome has generated controversy with the American Academy of Pediatrics posting this information online at healthychildren.org:

"Some parents say that the GFCF diet has lessened their child's symptoms. Research, however, has found little support for the GFCF diet and "leaky gut" theory. Several studies of the GFCF diet in children with ASDs (autism spectrum disorders) have shown that removing gluten and casein from a child's diet did not improve social skills or communication, nor did it help with sleep duration and activity levels. Even so, it's possible that some children with ASDs who have significant gastrointestinal problems may reap some benefits from the GFCF diet, especially if they, coincidentally, also have celiac disease (gluten-sensitivity autoimmune disorder).

"Still many parents try to remove gluten and casein from their child's diet. In fact, the GFCF diet is the most widely used CAM intervention (complementary and alternative medicine) among children who have ASDs. It's generally considered safe, and some parents report that diet has actually made a difference in their child's behavior. But it's hard to know if these behavioral changes are directly related to the GFCF diet or if they are the result of another intervention that the child may be undergoing at the same time."

Whether or not the syndrome actually exists, some benefits could be obtained from a gluten- and casein-free diet.

The Gluten-Free/Casein-Free Diet

Avoid

Grains That Contain Gluten

- Wheat
- Durum
- Bulgur
- Oats
- Rye
- Barley
- Millet
- Kamut
- Spelt

Products That Contain Gluten

- Adhesives
- Stickers
- Stamps
- Envelope glue
- Medications
- Vitamins
- Play-Doh
- Washing detergents
- Personal hygiene products
- Soaps, Shampoos
- Toothpaste
- Lip balms, Cosmetics

Foods That Contain Gluten

- Bread
- Pasta
- Cereals
- Cookies
- Crackers
- Vinegar
- Soups
- Sauces
- Seasonings
- Artificial coloring
- Spices
- Candy

Foods That Contain Casein

- Milk: Cow, Goat, Breast
- Butter
- Cheese
- Sour Cream
- Yogurt
- Ice Cream
- Margarine
- Soy Cheese

Speak to your doctor or nutritionist before starting the GFCF diet to reduce the risk of nutritional deficiency. Remember, when you remove something from the diet, you must replace the vitamins and minerals that will be lost in the process.

Autistic boys have thinner bones, according to information I have read on the Internet. Therefore, it would be essential to supplement calcium and vitamin D to support bone health when removing dairy from the diet. A GFCF diet can be difficult and somewhat expensive. I believe anyone contemplating the diet should be tested for Leaky Gut, celiac disease, and wheat and dairy allergies, before embarking on this adventure.

After all, I know we have our hands full and don't need added stress to deal with. As a small step, try starting with gluten then casein elimination to know which one or maybe both, are or are not causing stomach and/or behavioral problems. It is important to give your trial approximately three months to see if your child reaps any benefits.

Marilyn Le Breton, the mother of an autistic son and author of *Diet Intervention and Autism: Implementing the Gluten Free and Casein Free Diet for Autistic Children and Adults: A Practical Guide for Parents,* takes the GFCF diet a step further. She suggests eliminating MSG and aspartame

CHAPTER 28

The Gaps Diet & Natasha McBride, M.D.

Since our children differ in many ways, it's important for us to uncover what works for our child and what does not. This short overview of the GAPS diet (Gut and Psychology Syndrome) outlines another dietary approach to reducing the effect of autism.

Hippocrates said, "All diseases begin in the gut." The GAPS diet contends that if you heal the gut, you heal what ails you. Natasha Campbell McBride says her diet is not a way of life; it's for a specific period of time, to heal the gut and restore its flora. McBride, a neurologist practicing in England, is the mother of an autistic son whom she says she has recovered, declaring him, "off the autistic spectrum."

The GAPS diet holds that food that is not digested becomes toxic which leads to disease. Healing the digestive disorders will heal the psychological issues that arise because of those disorders.

Gut dysbiosis or microbial imbalances in the gut lead to autism, ADD (Attention Deficit Disorder), depression, and schizophrenia, according to McBride. By eliminating food sensitivities and repairing the gut with probiotics, digestive enzymes, omega-3s, and zinc, health can be restored to the gut in three months.

Patients avoid starch and sugars for two years. Wheat, sugar, processed foods, and all additives will have to be out for much longer.

Eating fermented foods with each meal will help you digest without digestive enzyme supplements. The best foods for the person on the GAPS diet are eggs, meat and fish—fresh or frozen. Fruit should be eaten raw, alone and separately from meals. Have plenty of natural fats in every meal. Balanced pH is important. All protein foods, such as meats, fish, eggs, and cheese leave an acid ash in the body. Vegetables are alkalizing, so combine protein with vegetables. Apple cider vinegar is very alkalizing; drink it daily by adding one teaspoon of cider vinegar to every glass of water you drink. Fermented foods are also alkalizing. Avoid processed foods. Do not use microwave to warm food; use a conventional oven or stove.

Foods to Avoid

- Sugar
- Aspartame
- Alcoholic beverages except wine
- Tinned and processed foods
- Grains
- Breakfast cereals
- Starchy vegetables (potatoes, parsnips, yam, artichoke, sweet potato)
- Milk
- Fruit juices except freshly pressed
- Beans except navy beans and green beans
- Coffee and strong tea
- Soft drinks
- Anything with colors, preservative, flavoring and other chemicals including soy.

Recommended Foods

Buy fresh or frozen meat, fish, or shellfish, not smoked, salted, or preserved in any way. You need to eat gelatinous meats every day. Eat all the fats on the meat. Lean meat will not be good. Liver and organ meats should be eaten on a regular basis.

Eggs two or three a day, yolks eaten raw; although this is controversial because of salmonella concerns.

Fresh vegetables, apart from starchy veggies, stew with plenty of garlic, added at the end of cooking.

Fresh fruit must be ripe and eaten between meals.

Avocado. Make sure it's ripe. Serve with meals.

Butter is better than substitutes.

Coconut oil and palm oil very good for cooking.

Cold pressed olive oil for salads.

Nuts and seeds bought just shelled—not roasted, salted, coated, or processed in any way. Almond flour is available to bake with. Almond milk for your child who likes milk.

Replace table salt with unprocessed salt, such as Celtic salt or Himalayan crystal salt.

Garlic will normalize gut flora and stimulate the immune system. Try to eat a whole head every day.

Unprocessed honey is the only sweetener allowed. In baking, use dried fruit.

There you have it: excerpts from the GAPS diet. For more information go to www.GutAndPsychologySyndrome.com. A special thank you to the McBrides for granting permission to share this information with my readers.

Comments

Controversy exists regarding concentrations of lead in the bone broth suggested in the preliminary diet. Also be cautious with raw egg yolks because of salmonella. Most all other suggestions are tenets of healthy, clean eating that is good for all of us. Lastly, be aware that mothers may pop their corks over limiting their microwave use and alcoholic consumption. And be careful when sending your child out to socialize after feeding him or her a whole head of garlic!

For all of you who would do anything possible to help your child, be careful not to burn out. Proven methods will be helpful. New diets may or may not reap benefits for your child. That's why I suggested testing to see if your child has sensitivities or Leaky Gut to begin with. If your family is in a particularly stressful time don't take on something that may throw you over the edge. Also, you can try diet modification, instead of a wholesale change. Try eating organic whenever possible, fresh foods instead of canned, and cut out soda, excess sugar, and processed foods, to start. We all know these things will make for a healthier way of eating. Then, at some time if feeling brave or bored (ha-ha), you can try the GAPS diet. Remember Dr. McBride recovered her son and attributes this diet to that process. As parents, we sometimes need to turn over every stone; sometimes it's just a matter of timing.

These excerpts are not intended to replace reading Dr. McBride's book. They are intended for educational purposes to let you know what's being published in hopes of recovering your child.

CHAPTER 29

Steps To Health: Pesticides and Antibiotics, Flame Retardants, Lotions & Potions, Clean Food, Clean Air, and Green Home

As I mentioned earlier, I have included some of my research from my own book, *How I Saved My Own Life and You Can Too*!

I am finally able to make the connection between cancer and autism = toxic overload. Therefore, I believe some of the protocol I mentioned in my previous book needs to be included here:

Pesticides and Antibiotics

Breast cancer incidence may be linked to both pesticide exposure and overuse of antibiotics.

We know now that overuse of antibiotics creates holes in the intestines causing "Leaky Gut." That will unleash a wide host of problems in our autistic children.

"Pesticides are so lethal that a chemist who swallowed an infinitesimal dose, amounting to 0.00424 of an ounce, was instantaneously paralyzed and died before he could take an antidote he had prepared in advance and had at hand," John Robbins, author of *Diet for a New America: How Your Food Choices Affect Your Health, Happiness, the Future of Life on Earth,* and other books.

How many of you believe that washing your fruits and vegetables keeps you safe from pesticides? Did you know most pesticides in the diet come from meat and dairy? How many moms wash the apples they give to their youngsters and then serve them a glass of pesticide-laden milk? How does this happen?

"Cows are kept in deplorable farm conditions. They are so filthy and crowded together that animals get sick. Then they are given antibiotics and dipped in a bath of toxic pesticides. These pesticides are retained in the fat of the animal. The cows become carriers of the most deadly chemicals ever known." (John Robbins)

From *Diet for a New America*

"Dioxin is by far the most toxic chemical known to mankind. Created as a manufacturing by-product from processes such as waste incineration, chemical and pesticide manufacturing, and pulp and paper bleaching, it is an environmental and organic pollutant.

"Millions of pounds of this lethal chemical have been sprayed on the land in the United States. Cows, pigs, and chickens contain in their flesh the dioxin residues from all the plants they have ever eaten." (Robbins)

"Humans who eat beef...can get a concentrated dose of dioxin that has built up from years." (Lewis Regenstein, author of *How to Survive in America the Poisoned*)

Dioxin causes cancer, birth defects (possibly autism, miscarriages, and death in lab animals at the lowest possible levels to test—one part per trillion.

How many pregnant women eat steak, hamburger, chicken, and bacon when they are carrying their child!

Heptachlor

Several years after an insecticide containing heptachlor was finally banned in the United States, the U.S Department of Agriculture discovered that, as part of its school lunch program, it had sent 40,000 pounds of heptachlor-contaminated, ground pork to schools in Louisiana and Arkansas. By the time they realized what had been done, over 14,000 pounds of poisoned pork had been consumed by the children.

The problem with pesticides is the damage and havoc they create lasts over time. When we eat bacteria, we get sick immediately and can quickly experience cramps, vomiting, and fever. When we consume pesticides, they accumulate gradually over time and we get chilling effects, such as cancer and autism, many years later.

PCBs

"Monsanto Corporation first produced PCBs (polychlorinated biphenyls) in the United States in the 1930s. They were used to manufacture less flammable cooling and insulating fluids for industrial transformers and capacitors and flexible coating for electrical wiring and electric components.

"Monsanto had a motto: 'Without chemicals, life itself would be impossible.' Not long after PCBs were introduced, it became apparent these chemicals posed major problems for human beings. Three years after production began, the faces and bodies of 24 out of 24 workers in the Monsanto plant became disfigured. But that didn't stop Monsanto; since then more than 750,000 tons of these deadly poisons have been produced. They can be found today in every river in America, the snow in Antarctica, and probably the tissues in every single fish in the waters of this planet." (Robbins)

So there you have it! We eat fish, we get PCBs. We eat beef, we get dioxin. We eat pork, we get heptachlor poisoning. And all the time, the government is reassuring us our food supply is safe!

Even when these pesticides are banned in the United States, they are then sold to third-world countries. These countries use the dangerous chemicals on their products and then we import their beef for our fast food restaurants.

Mother's Milk

We all know breastfeeding is good for our babies, isn't it? Not really!

Even mother's milk is contaminated with dangerous pesticides and toxins consumed and accumulated by the mother. If the truth be known: mother's milk is so polluted that if it were made into a product for sale on the global market, it could not be shipped or transported across state lines because it would qualify as a hazardous substance. What can be done?

Minimize your intake of meat, fish, dairy, and eggs. Choose organic foods. Reduce your intake of imported foods, like coffee, sugar, tea, and bananas, because farmers in other countries such as Costa Rica, Ecuador, Guatemala, and Mexico use much greater concentrations of pesticides than even American agriculture allows. Choose in-season, locally grown fruits and vegetables. And remember, the worst of all foods are fast food hamburgers, because they are often made from beef imported from Central America.

I highly recommend the book by John Robbins, *Diet for a New America*, if you want to learn more about your food supply.

Dr. Oz Strikes Again

Our beloved doctor and wonderfully informed TV personality has provided yet another supersonic show!

As I'm just about to wrap up the book and send the manuscript up to the editor, I got a glimpse of something about flame retardants. It seems flame retardants are everywhere and not to our benefit. Eighty percent of upholstered furniture contains these toxic chemicals. Flame retardants cause:

- Thyroid disorders
- Birth defects
- Diminished IQ
- Hyperactivity
- Infertility
- Cancer

What's even worse: **they don't work as promised**. The Dr. Oz show simulated a burning cushion with and without retardants; the difference was not significant enough to warrant such health dangers.

Flame-retardants are a scheme by the tobacco industry and big chemical companies to make money and protect themselves. People were dying in fires caused by cigarettes. Therefore, to avoid lawsuits and in an attempt to protect themselves, the tobacco industry said, in effect, "It's not our problem, you should make furniture that is cigarette resistant."

Hence, flame retardant furniture became a reality because of that nonsense and the efforts of the **Citizens for Fire Safety**—which lobbied for flame retardants in all flammable products, including crib mattresses and children's car seats. But Citizens for Fire Safety are not our citizens; the group consists of the three largest makers of chemical flame-retardants, of course!

Tests on Children's Furniture

Recent laboratory tests were conducted on children's furniture, pillows, car seats, and other materials, as well as urine samples from the mothers and children using the furniture. The results were not good. All pieces of furniture sampled had toxic flame-retardants in them. Moms and children tested positive for flame-retardants in their urine. Some samples were alarmingly high.

Heather Stapleton, an environmental researcher at Duke University, can hardly keep up with the demand for testing samples from the concerned public.

To reduce inhaling flame retardants, dust and mop frequently, plus vacuum with HEPA (high-efficiency particulate absorption) filters. Wash your hands and your child's often and always before eating.

Buy upholstered furniture with cotton, wool, or polyester fiberfill instead of foam.

Most of us are angry about this dilemma, but we need to be proactive on this subject. Always check labels for flame-retardants or flame-resistant products.

Hope for the Future

In 2013, California Governor Jerry Brown changed the mandate that furniture has to have these chemicals. So in 2014, the consumer will have a choice to buy furniture that is safe.

Toxic Lotions and Potions

Let's begin with the moms. We need to be in the best health possible to take care of a special needs child.

On the jacket cover of Andrew Wakefield's book *Callous Disregard*, I was shocked to see this admission from a very frightened, truthful mother.

> Do not judge me too harshly Dr. Wakefield but when I die I am taking my son with me. You see, I'm all he has. I'm the only one who loves him.
>
> —A mother's plea

So you moms out there, we need to live as long as possible to fulfill our mission of recovering our children. That's why we need to check our lotions and potions and be aware of radiation hazards for both you and your family.

How many of you believe your cosmetics are safe? The FDA must be on top of poisons in our potions, wouldn't you think? Well, think again; a little-known fact is that there are only 10 ingredients banned from cosmetics in the United States. Ingredients banned from cosmetics in the European Union number over one thousand. . . shocking. . . hair raising!

Every day many of us use multiple "beauty products," starting with our shampoo, deodorant, moisture lotion, and finally, makeup. We sometimes think that expensive products are made from superior ingredients. That is not necessarily true. My favorite Chanel lipstick rated a 6 on a scale from 1 to 10, with 10 being most toxic; that is not good. Literally, I was ingesting this almost every day. I remember a few years back I saw a curious picture in a magazine of a soup bowl with broken lipsticks floating in it. I thought at the time, it was interesting. I recognized the fact we ingest our lipsticks, but I didn't realize how toxic they might be. Some of your favorite drugstore brands scored the unspeakable number 9 on the toxicity chart.

According to Skin Deep, an online cosmetic safety database maintained by the nonprofit Environmental Working Group, all cosmetics could be rated from 0–10, with 0–2 low hazard, 3–6 moderate, and 7–10 high risk.

Every time our bottle of liquid makeup runs dry we run to purchase another one. Where does that stuff go? The skin drinks it and it enters our bodies, so it's not surprising harmful chemicals have gotten into our breast milk and children as well. These chemicals cause cancer, birth defects, learning disabilities, and a host of other health problems that plague our society today. The cosmetics industry assures us that toxins in our cosmetics are safe, but since no government standard for safety exists, companies can say whatever they want about the safety of their products. The cosmetic industry says the amounts are allowable and small. Yet, most of us ladies use many products every day. Over time, the cumulative exposure builds up and can result in illness.

According to Skin Deep, product categories of highest concern are: hair color, hair bleach, hair relaxer, nail polish, and skin lighteners. A word about skin lighteners: Many dermatologists give their patients hydroquinone for brown spots; but just because many do so does not make it safe. As a matter of fact, hydroquinone is a possible carcinogen and probable neurotoxin, and can also cause irreversible skin disease.

Some chemicals are known to be toxic but are still in our cosmetics: Mercury is in eye drops and mascara; lead is in hair dyes and cleaners; and dioxin, from the breakdown of petrochemicals such as mineral oil, paraffin, and petroleum, is found in hair relaxers, anti-aging creams, perfumes, makeup foundations, lipstick, and lip balm. Nanoparticles of these harmful substances are capable of being absorbed directly into the bloodstream from eye shadows, bronzers, sunscreens, and lotions.

The word "natural" is no guarantee the product is safe. According to Skin Deep, Neutrogena's after-sun treatment with natural soy has one of the highest hazard ratings of the lotions tested. Neutrogena®, owned by the global corporation Johnson & Johnson, markets its products as superior because of their "natural" ingredients and recommendations from health-care providers. I was using a Neutrogena product myself. I thought it was a good product because it was recommended by the American Cancer Society. The product, Neutrogena Ultra Sheer Dry Touch Sunblock SPF 55, scored a 7, equaling a health hazard. How ironic, a product that is pricey, feels good on the skin, and is recommended by the American Cancer Society is toxic.

The American Cancer Society evaluated the product from a UVA and UVB perspective. It does block harmful sunrays, which helps prevent skin cancer and melanoma. But the big picture is not good.

Ingredients in many sunscreens have raised concerns about reproductive toxicity and irritation to skin, eyes, or lungs. I stopped using the product immediately and returned it to the pharmacy where I purchased it. If you want SPF protection use a safe sunscreen such as California Babies and others. Look for a white residue when you apply it. That's the zinc oxide or titanium dioxide that you need for safe protection. I began to see how all the lotions and potions I was using were like taking liquid gels of them daily. We all know these products are for external use only. Now we know they enter our skin as surely as if we had swallowed them…yuck!

So, if you won't drink or eat the product, don't put it on your skin or your precious child.

To reiterate, children with autism most likely have methylation problems. They do not clear toxins properly. Therefore, live in a "green home." Filter your drinking water. No VOC paint, VOC glue, carpeting and pressed board furniture, paraffin candles, conventional room fresheners. Limit chlorine: cleaning products, swimming pools, and long showers. Air out your home daily;

the air inside is twice as polluted as the outside air. This happens from "off-gassing" that occurs when products release toxic fumes into the air, such as particleboard cabinets, formaldehyde from room sprays and carpets, and other substances such as toxic cleaning products and pest removal poisons. Do not allow dust and mold to gather in your home.

Eat Clean Food

Eat organic foods whenever possible. Avoid artificial colors that can agitate our kids and cause more suffering. Many mothers will have to test for allergies and avoid those triggers: gluten and dairy.

Avoid sodas. Do not store or cook your food in plastic containers. Avoid fast foods and processed foods. Be especially vigilant when it comes to fast food burgers!

Cut down on refined sugars. Sugar can encourage cancer cells to grow, yeast to proliferate, and obesity to develop in our children. Too much sugar can lead to the "Leaky Gut Syndrome" mentioned earlier.

Do eat lots of colorful fruits and vegetables. Drink lots of water. Take vitamins and supplements to maintain a healthy body and mind.

SULFORAPHANE

One such vegetable and supplement is getting a lot of attention in 2014. Broccoli sprouts containing the compound sulforaphane are being studied with regards to helping individuals with ASD. Although studies have been small to date, the results are promising. Sulforaphane derived from broccoli sprouts helped ease autism symptoms in nearly half of the 29 individuals enrolled in a small 18-week trial. Doses range from 50 to 150umol daily depending on weight. Liver inflammation may result. Therefore, at this time if you choose to go ahead with a trial it is very important to work closely with a physician to monitor possible side effects. I am sure we will be hearing a lot more about this subject in the near future.

Install air filters and plants in your child's bedroom. Beware of secondhand smoke! Live in an area of town that has less pollution, like the suburbs if possible, surrounded by trees. Remove carpeting; rid your home of mold and dust mites as much as possible. Place those stuffed animals in the dryer often to remove dust mites.

CHAPTER 30

Radiation Risks

X-Ray Hazards

Many people instinctually back away from an X-ray machine and do not stay in the same room with their children when they are X-rayed. Why do we do this??? Because we all know radiation exposure is not good for you.

Every time I express concern over X-ray exposure, the technician or doctor will assure me the risk is miniscule. The problem with their reassurance is neither knows how many X-rays or scans I have already had. Radiation exposure is cumulative. When you fill out paperwork in a doctor's office, he or she is very certain to ask you about all your preview surgeries and medications you are taking. Never has a doctor asked me about an X-ray or scan diary to ascertain the amount of radiation I have been exposed to. Now that I am in my 50s, they are even less concerned. Why is that? If a person gets exposed to a carcinogen it takes usually 20 or 30 years to cause cancer. It is assumed that if I were to get an overdose of radiation from scans at this age, I would not manifest a fatal disease until my 70s or 80s. Somehow this information is not comforting. Most of us would agree that we would rather die in our sleep in our 90s!

CT Scans

I became even more concerned after reading a Sept. 7, 2008, article in the *Los Angeles Times*, "Revolutionary (CT) scans come with a risk." The article explained that computed tomography (CT) scans were introduced in the 1970s and have become a standard procedure, with U.S. doctors ordering 68.7 million CT scans (in 2007), more than triple the number in 1995!

The article went on to explain that this increase is causing rising concern that more frequent use of radiation is negatively affecting the health of our nation.

The article, a study published in the *New England Journal of Medicine*, estimated that CT scans administered today could cause up to 2% of cancer deaths in two or three decades. I believe that even a tiny exposure spread over a large population can add up to tens of thousands of cancer deaths every year.

Cancer Risk

CT scans can create cancer risks when:

- Radiation loosens an electron from an atom, which creates an ion that damages a cell's DNA
- The dose of radiation is insufficient to kill the irradiated cells and the damaged cells divide and multiply over time, spreading the faulty genetic information. "The Result is Cancer," the article concluded.

The best data on low-level radiation exposure come from studies of 25,000 survivors from two or three miles outside the blast zone of Hiroshima and Nagasaki, on which atomic bombs were dropped at the end of WW II. The residents of those cities received between five and 150milliverts—the equivalent of a few CT scans—a small but statistically significant increase in cancer and death rates was noted, according to studies.

Even scarier was what followed: a conclusion by the National Academy of Sciences that no safe level of radiation exposure exists and that even small doses pose some health risks.

CT scans have become an economic consideration for doctors and hospitals, the article continued, with Siemens and General Electric Company promoting their easy profitability. Two scans a day can pay for the device in five years. Ten scans a day can bring in more than $400,000 a year profit, according to the *Times* article.

"Patients come in with a headache," Dr. Scott Lederhaus, a neurosurgeon in Pomona, was quoted in the article. "If they don't get scanned and something gets missed, they can sue. So I order the scan, it's not worth the aggravation."

"Since doctors have been suffering as the dollars and cents are being squeezed out of a medical practice, why shouldn't they get their own equipment?" Dr. Madyoon, another cardiologist in the article, asked. "You've got to survive."

A report by the U.S. Government Accountability Office suggested that financial concerns for doctors were a major factor in the rising number of CT scans. It is natural for a doctor to use machines they purchased or have some stake in. These doctors are two to seven times more likely to order tests than other doctors who made referrals to outside facilities.

The standard unit of measure for radiation dose exposure is millisieverts. A CT scan delivers a dose of 5 to 25millisieverts. The United States limits public exposure to 1millisievert per year, although 50millisieverts is the allowable exposure for those working in radiation environments. According to the *Times* article, one doctor who surveyed records for an imaging company discovered that 11,535 patients had received more than 50millisieverts from CT scans, 107 patients had received more than 200millisieverts, and one poor soul got 992millisieverts! After doing the research, I began thinking about all the X-rays and scans that I have had. Every one of those times I was reassured that the radiation dose was nothing to worry about.

A CT scan to my left axilla (underarm) to image a swollen lymph node, a complete bone scan with radioactive isotopes to rule out bone cancer. I was having aches and pains in my joints from fibromyalgia, so a complete body scan was needed. Remember when they were the rage?? The tech actually told me that all the employees in the office were going to have one a year.

I also had a CT scan of my lungs just a year ago because my gynecologist suggested I have my lungs checked because of my age. Now I realize because of my age, that CT scan could have started a lung cancer in progress. I was given a barium enema, somewhere along the way, to view my large intestine (I have a family history of polyps). I read that one researcher concluded higher cancer risks are attributed to barium enemas.

Young girls who have had X-ray for lung infections have a higher risk later in life to develop breast cancer, some doctor's say.

I can't go back and undo what has been done, but I am wiser now. I will always be hyper vigilant about CT scans in the future and have one only if it is truly necessary.

We must always be cognizant of the fact we are raising little canaries. Our children are more susceptible to toxics, we know now. Maybe they are more sensitive to radiation? A little may do a lot of damage.

So, when you go to your dentist, don't give in to yearly or biannual full mouth films. Your child can do with much less than that. Mouth cancer is on the rise in this country; it just might be from all the dental X-rays we have been exposed to.

Last week, I was coming home from Europe. At the airport I was faced with the scan machine. I waited to see if I would be selected to go through the scan. Sometimes, only a few "random individuals" are asked to go through the scan. This time everyone was given the pleasure to have a turn. I immediately stepped aside and refused. I also refused for my son Jon, who was behind me. A large woman gave me a disgusted look and told me to stand on the side to wait for a pat down. While we were waiting for security to arrive, a woman checking baggage called me over. She said, "You're doing the right thing for yourself and especially your son. I wouldn't trust the government to tell the truth about these scanners."

I thought to myself, I'm not sure about any of this radiation stuff, so I will err on the side of safety.

My dentist recently said to me, "Ann, you haven't had a full set of X-rays for 10 years. If you resist any longer, I will not be able to treat you."

I left and immediately started looking for another dentist!

One last word about the dentist, don't let them put silver amalgams in your child's teeth. They may tell you they are only baby teeth, so it doesn't matter, it does matter. Silver amalgams are 50% mercury by weight. Every time you child brushes their teeth, eats something hot or cold, gets their teeth cleaned, it accelerates mercury vapors that end up in their bloodstream or mucus membranes. Then, it will be stored and will poison your child.

CHAPTER 31

The Vaccine Controversy

The vaccine controversy can fill a whole book. This section is not meant to be definitive but simply provide a sampling of the research, information, and points of view surrounding this subject.

It's no secret Jenny McCarthy believes vaccinations caused her son's autism. So strong are her convictions, Jenny wrote the forward to *Callous Disregard: Autism and Vaccines—The Truth Behind a Tragedy* by Andrew Wakefield.

> "I'm so glad Andy Wakefield has the chance to tell his story...I believe
> Dr. Wakefield is the kind of doctor and scientist who will ultimately help us
> end the epidemic of children with autism...I believe history will be kind to
> Andy Wakefield. He will be seen as a man that stood up for truth, despite extreme pressure to stand down." Jenny McCarthy (excerpts)
>
> April 22, 2010

Strong faith and words in support of Andrew Wakefield. But the online information available on *Wikipedia*, "MMR vaccine controversy" tells a different story.

According to the article online, the measles, mumps, rubella (MMR) controversy in 1998 was caused by a fraudulent research paper published in *The Lancet* by Dr. Andrew Wakefield. The charges by *The Sunday Times* of London journalist Brian Deer were conflicts of interest on Wakefield's part, manipulation of evidence, and broken ethical codes. In May 2010, Wakefield was found guilty by the General Medical Council of Medical Malpractice, which keeps a list of medical practitioners in the UK, and was struck off the Medical Register. Wakefield could no longer practice as a doctor.

"The scientific consensus is that no evidence links the vaccine to the development of autism, and that the vaccine's benefits greatly outweigh its risks," the online article reads. Because of this debacle, the National Vaccine Injury Compensation Program denied the claims of injury brought by parents of autistic children in the United States.

Another theory on autism blames industrial pollution and other toxins. Yet, an online article entitled "Why Don't the Amish Get Autism?" found on Examiner.com notes that many Amish live within the heavily polluted and industrial northeast. Therefore, the Amish throw a heavy wrench into the "industrial pollution" theory. But the article adds that the Amish do practice healthy lifestyles, which includes, high regard for clean and safe foods, and they also do not vaccinate their children, practices which have changed within the Amish population over the years so that few conclusions can be drawn from their situation.

Meanwhile, in Italy in 2012, an Italian court awarded damages to the parents of a now autistic child, concluding that they had demonstrated beyond a reasonable doubt that the disease was caused by the MMR vaccine.

Further, these excerpts from *Healing and Preventing Autism*, by McCarthy and Jerry Kartzinel, M.D., provide food for thought about mercury poisoning from vaccines:

Jenny: Everyone believes it was completely removed from vaccines, which isn't true. It was only reduced.

Dr. Jerry: We have to understand that it's well accepted that mercury is one of the most toxic substances known to man on this planet. So, how can they justify even a small amount of mercury to a pregnant woman in the form of a flu shot or in giving it to a newborn in the hepatitis B?

Dr. Kartzinel explains even though mercury has been reduced in vaccines, it is still a deadly toxin even in exquisitely small amounts. You don't need anything but a very small amount to do damage.

Jenny: In 2002, the manufacturers changed the formulations of the contents of vaccines, namely decreasing thimerosal and increasing aluminum. Then they added the flu shot to the vaccine schedule, which has mercury in it. Are they stupid? Wait, of course they are!

Healing and Preventing Autism, states that the rate of autism has increased with the increase of vaccinations. Ten vaccinations were required in 1983 and the autism rate was one in 10,000 people. With 36 vaccinations required in 2008, the autism rate is now one in 150!

I highly recommend you read *Healing and Preventing Autism* by McCarthy and Dr. Kartzinel. It's an amazing book that's bound to give you pieces to your puzzle in recovering your child.

If I've whet your appetite for asking more questions or taking a stand one way or the other about vaccination, then I did my job.

What I learned along the way is that many shades of gray exist on this issue. It is important to vaccinate your child, in my opinion, but maybe we need to cut back to a less aggressive vaccination schedule. It might be prudent to space the shots, instead of giving so many at once. Parents must demand complete removal of mercury from all required vaccinations. It is most important to protect our children's safety, not the profits of the drug manufacturers!

CHAPTER 32

Exercise Benefits for Autism—Reducing Negative Behaviors: Aerobics, Swimming, Martial Arts, and Horse Riding

Aerobic Exercise

Persons with autism often engage in self-stimulating behavior such as body rocking, spinning, hand flapping, head-nodding, object tapping, gazing at lights, and mouthing, or putting objects into their mouths. Research has shown that this interferes with performance of positive social behaviors and learning and presents problems for integration into mainstream education classes.

Research on aerobic exercise has shown that it can decrease these negative behaviors without decreasing other positive behaviors. Specifically, use of aerobics with students in various special populations has been shown to reduce aggressive behavior and unproductive and disruptive behavior, plus improves work performance and on-task behavior.

Fitness professional Dylan Drobish, in his online article, "How Exercise Benefits Autism Spectrum Disorders," examines how physical activity can help transform the lives of people with atypical brains. Drobish writes:

". . . While people with autism spectrum disorders tend to be less physically active than their neurotypical peers (even when they are sufficiently capable of performing the motor tasks involved), recent research has uncovered some remarkable benefits that can be attained by

ASD individuals participating in regular exercise..

"A 2010 review by Lang et al. that examined physical activity interventions for ASD participants noted significant decrease in stereotypy, aggression, and off-task behavior among the 64 participants. In addition, participants showed improvements in on-task behavior, academic engagement, and appropriate motor behavior following vigorous exercise. A similar review by Sowa and Meulenbroek also found improvements in social functioning when participants were provided with an individualized exercise program. . ."

Drobish continues with a section called "How Exercise Heals the Brain," in which he writes "Some studies have found that, in people with ASD, the amygdala and hippocampus are reduced in size compared to the total brain volume, and this likely reflects the underdevelopment of the neural connections of limbic structures with other parts of the brain, particularly the cortex. . . While we won't know with any certainty until further studies are conducted, it may be possible that growth of new cells in the hippocampus and the modulation of existing connections in the prefrontal cortex—an area heavily involved in attention, planning, impulse control, and even empathy—is responsible for improvements in function exhibited by ASD individuals that exercise.

"One specific area whose function seems to be altered in autism spectrum disorders is the anterior cingulate gyrus, which helps the brain shift its attention to adapt to change when needed. Given the restricted, repetitive behaviors of many autistic individuals, as well as a general resistance toward change or unexpected circumstances, the involvement of this area is indeed likely. Changes have also been observed in this area in response to physical exercise. . . ".

Another article from which I have extracted useful paragraphs is "On Autism and Exercise" written by Daniel Hawthorne, who himself has high functioning autism and has written a book, *A Reason for Hope: Insights into Autism.*

"Someone once asked me what, if anything, I would do differently as principal of a school for autistic children. I responded that I would have the children out running and playing vigorously for at least an hour twice a day. . . It's my heart-felt conviction that physical activity of some kind is vital to helping autistic children, like me at one time, function."

Hawthorne's experience and feelings have been validated in the connection that has been found between physical activity and the development of new nerves in the hippocampus. The hippocampus of autistic children tends to be smaller than "neurotypicals." Even "brain exercises" can enlarge the hippocampus and help our autistic children function more typically.

Hawthorne continues, "My point is this: Autistic children need physical activity to help them develop as well as to help them deal with high levels of frustration from sensory difficulties. I would even say the body craves it. (Emphasis mine) I believe that diet and drugs have their place in treating autism, but so does aerobic activity."

Swimming and Horse Riding

Swimming is also therapeutic for children with autism as the excerpts from this online article, "Autism and Swimming: Children with Autism Can Benefit From Physical Activity."

"The Children with autism are certainly not incapable of participating in athletics. Just ask 16-year-old Nathan of Central Indiana if he lets autism slow him down. He actively participates as a member of his high school swim team . . .

". . . 'People with autism experience levels of sensory perception that most of us wouldn't know or understand,' Dr. John O'Connor said. 'It overloads them, so they engage in behaviors that distract them. Exercise gives them the same benefits but it doesn't have the negative social connotations.'

"John O'Connor, associate professor of adapted physical education at Montana State University—Northern, explained why. Running and swimming involve rhythmic movements that are similar to stereotypical behaviors and may distract people with autism the same way flapping their hands or walking on their toes does . . .

". . . Swim instructor Julie Gross of the Super Swimmers Foundation . . . has witnessed how swimming can help an [autistic] child to improve their speech, coordination, and physical fitness with an activity as simple and enjoyable as swimming."

The full article (http://superswimmersfoundation.org/Autism-and-Swimming.htm) also contains links to other information on swimming and autism, including:

- Enhancing mental development through swimming
- Increasing intelligence and healing the mind through exercise
- Mr. Blue and his crew support surfers for autism
- Swimming accesses the five pathways to the brain
- Swim lessons for the autistic child
- The Super Swimmers Foundation

I also found information about horse riding in this online article, "Positive Impacts of Exercise for Children with Autism," by Elyse Morin, an undergraduate student in the College of Health and Human Performance, University of Florida.

"Horse riding, or Hippotherapy, is an exercise that offers benefits ranging from the therapeutic effects of the repetitive movement of the horse's gait, to the gradual social interaction that it provides to the rider. As the child rides, he is able to create a relationship with the horse as he is calmed by the sensory feedback that he is getting from the movement of the horse's hips as it walks. He is also able to create relationships with the instructor, therapist, and volunteers, and possibly other riders. This exercise is generally nonverbal, and allows for the child to interact with the horse and others without anxieties caused by their social and communicative deficits."

Dancing

If you thought dancing was just a pleasurable pastime, ask the celebrities on TV's *Dancing with the Stars* if they got a workout! For kids with autism who may be averse to traditional exercise, here's a fun way for them to move. The online article, *"Dancing Can Benefit Individuals with Autism,"* was posted May 11, 2011 by Susan Moffitt.

"After the stunning performance of James Hobley, the 11-year-old with autism who blew away the audience on *Britain's Got Talent* with an amazing dance routine, it's a fitting time to address the benefits of dance for children on the autistic spectrum.

"The practice of dance is highly structured and very ritualized, a selling point for children with autism. Dance has the power to unlock the imagination of a concrete thinker and it empowers the dancer to give expression to their inner life, something crucial to children who struggle with other modalities of communication . . .

". . . The combination of music and dance help the brain reorganize itself. In dance, the child processes music, learns movement, performs movement to that music, and then repeats it multiple times. The hearing, listening, processing, executing, and repetition enable a child's brain to forge new pathways, engaging both the right and left side of the brain.

"One form of dance therapy, The Feldenkrais method, deliberately focuses on the interplay between the right and left hemispheres . . .

" . . . Above all else, dance is fun and should be approached in that spirit. As someone with a degree in dance and decades of experience, I do recommend making sure a child's dance teacher is always warm and supportive. There's many a petty tyrant in tights who can potentially be damaging to a child psychologically. Additionally, watch closely for eating disorders (a prime occupational hazard for dancers)."

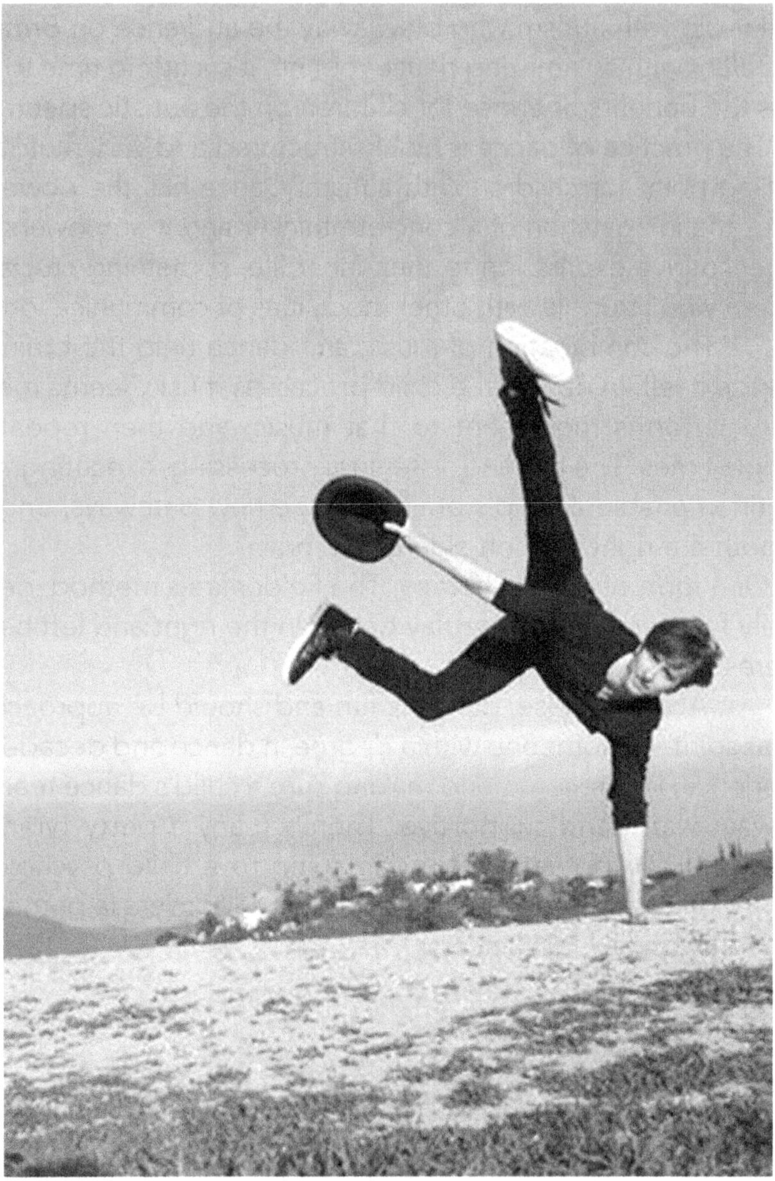

JON DOING HIS BEST IMITATION OF MICHAEL JACKSON

Martial Arts and Autism

Parents and instructors have observed that martial arts provide enormous benefits. Children with autism are encouraged to come out of their shells. They become more social and cooperative. Respect, honor, and humility are required in the dojo, values that will serve our children well in life.

The training of katas and rapid hand movements in conjunction with aerobic exercise helps the brain form new connections. Martial arts improve balance, hand-eye coordination, and eye contact in autistic students. Intensive exercise releases pent up energy in a socially appropriate manner. The dojo provides a sense of belonging and new friendships, all of which are priceless.

CHAPTER 33

Reversing Autism—The Genetic Challenge

Most of this book has been about causes, prevention, and therapies for autism, but research is also being done on ways to physically engineer changes. Fascinating! See the excerpt below from *Popular Science*, contained in their "Frontiers of Medicine: Radical Cures" feature story, posted 3/2/2010 by Corey Binns.

"Reversing Autism

". . . Mike Bear's mice weren't well. They were aggressive, slow learners, and kept convulsing into seizures—classic signs of Fragile X syndrome. But when the Massachusetts Institute of Technology neuroscientist tweaked a single receptor in the mice's brains, they began acting as if they had never been sick. Now he plans to do the same for people

"Fragile X syndrome, a genetic mutation on the X chromosome, is the most common source of inherited mental impairment, affecting one in every 4,000 boys and one in every 6,000 girls. It's also the most common cause of autism . . . Currently, the only drugs available for the syndrome treat the overt symptoms, such as anxiety and aggression. Bear's drug works at the syndrome's physical source.

"While studying mice, he learned that the disease allows a neuron's mGluR5 receptor to send out a flurry of signals telling the cell to produce protein. The protein overload causes a neuron to form many more connections to other neurons than normal, creating chaos by spreading nerve instructions to too many cells. Bear's drug, called STX107, inhibits the receptors to pare back the overproduction of proteins associated with Fragile X to a normal range . . . Bear says it could be a first step to treating other causes of autism."

So, there you have it. Even when it comes to something that used to seem impossible to change, like a mutation, there's hope. And that's the rainbow we might all be looking for.

CHAPTER 34

Is Everyone on the Spectrum? By Benjamin Wallace

"Is Everyone on the Autism Spectrum?" is a wonderful article by a very talented writer, Benjamin Wallace (no relation), published May 12, 2014, in *New York* magazine. I just had to include this in the closing chapters of the book.

Every era has its catchwords to describe non-typical behaviors. Recent ones include narcissistic, borderline, ice queen, attention deficit disordered, and so on. Recently Asperger syndrome has become the new catchall for husbands behaving badly or socially inappropriate behaviors by "typicals." Dismayingly, families raising children who are on the spectrum are sometimes told that they are lucky to have such geniuses among them. But the truth is that not all children with autism are geniuses and real hardships are involved in raising our children to be able to flourish. The Asperger movement has become so "socially special" that many people calling themselves Aspies are reluctant to give up the diagnosis, even though it has been dropped from the *DSM-5*, the *Diagnostic and Statistical Manual of Mental Disorders*, Fifth Edition, the U.S. authority for psychiatric diagnosis. Whatever you call a person on the spectrum, they are all struggling with mighty challenges.

It is not a joke as in "ass burgers" or an excuse for bad behavior, as Benjamin Wallace points out. I hope you find this article as interesting and enjoyable as I did.

Autism Spectrum: Are You On It?

If so, you're in good company. From Asperger's to "Asperger's," how the spectrum became quite so all-inclusive.

By Benjamin Wallace

"Is every man in America somewhere on it?" Nora Ephron wondered about the autism spectrum in an e-mail to a friend a few months before her death. "Is every producer on it? Is every 8-year-old boy who is obsessed with statistics on it? Sometimes, when we say someone is on the spectrum, do we just mean he's a prick? Or a pathological narcissist? I notice that at least three times a week I am told (or I tell someone) that some man or other is on the spectrum."

Ephron was hardly alone. In August, after a string of campaign-trail bloopers by Mitt Romney (e.g., at a New Hampshire parade, he described his lemonade as "lemon ... wet ... good"), noted diagnostician David Shuster, a television personality at Current TV, floated the idea that Romney might be on the spectrum. Shuster cited "an uncle who specializes in the field of Asperger's"—a mild variant of autism—who had "suggested that perhaps Mitt Romney has some sort of form of Asperger's because he's so socially inept in terms of being able to connect with people. What he thinks is funny is really sort of not so funny. I sort of wonder if there's some sort of tic or something that he has that's related to that."

Meanwhile, out on the Great Plains, one Dennis Stillings, writing in the Bismarck-based Dakota *Beacon* about Barack Obama, has adduced such telltale evidence as his "legendary clumsiness ... He has actually bowled a 37," "verbal glitches—possibly the reason for the ever-present teleprompters," and "infamous inability to relate" to arrive at a boldly contrarian thesis: "Obama may well not be narcissistic at all, but simply manifesting a typical feature of autism." Stillings then passes along the opinion of a friend of a friend "who actually works with autistic people" that the president of the United States "likely" has Asperger's, and speculates that this "may or may not be of significance" to the Obama administration's considerable funding of autism research.

The diagnosis is everywhere: Facebook's former head of engineering has stated that Mark Zuckerberg has "a touch of the Asperger's." *Time* suggested that the intensely awkward Bill Gates is autistic; a biographer of Warren Buffett wrote that the Oracle of Omaha, with his prodigious memory and "fascination with numbers," has "a vaguely autistic aura." On *Celebrity Rehab,* Dr. Drew Pinsky deemed Dennis Rodman (selectively hyperfocused, socially obtuse) a candidate for an Asperger's diagnosis, and the UCLA specialist brought in to make it official "seemed to concur," Pinsky told viewers. On the Asperger's community site Wrong Planet, threads like "Real life celebrities who have or probably have Asperger's" include Jim Carrey, Adolf Hitler, Daryl Hannah, Slash, Billy Joel, J.K. Rowling, and Adam Carolla, who makes the cut because "I've heard guests on his podcast remark on his lack of eye contact." "Kanye Probably Has Asperger's," BuzzFeed recently declared.

Still others are seeing it in themselves. David Byrne: "I was a peculiar young man—borderline Asperger's, I would guess." Craigslist founder Craig Newmark, noting his poor eye contact and limited social competency, blogged that Asperger's symptoms "feel uncomfortably familiar." Dan Harmon, the volatile creator of NBC's *Community,* told an interviewer last year that he had boned up on Asperger's symptoms when researching the character Abed: "The more I looked them up, the more familiar they seemed." Dan Aykroyd told NPR's Terry Gross that he was diagnosed with Asperger's as a child (a puzzling claim given that the diagnosis didn't exist prior to 1981, when Aykroyd turned 29); Aykroyd insisted he was being serious, and as evidence of his continuing symptoms he noted his "fascination with law enforcement and the police."

What is happening? What cultural through-line has emerged that would join such surreal-life bedfellows as a pop-piano-playing crooner, a flamboyant professional basketball player, a reclusive children's-book author, a twentysomething Internet gazillionaire, and a genocidal madman together in diagnostic brotherhood? How have we reached a point where partisans of left and right can regard the opposing candidates for the highest office in the land and see ... an arcane brain disorder? "It's an epidemic," Ephron wrote in her e-mail. "Or else a wildly over-diagnosed thing that there used to be other words for."

Every generation has its defining psychiatric malady, confidently diagnosed from afar by armchair non-psychiatrists. In the fifties, all those gray-suited organization men were married to "frigid" women. Until a few years ago, the country of self-obsessed boomers and reality-TV fame-seekers and vain politicians and bubble-riding Ponzi schemers made narcissistic personality disorder—diagnosis code 301.81 in the American Psychiatric Association's *Diagnostic and Statistical Manual of Mental Disorders,* fourth edition—the craziness of the moment. And who among us has not proudly copped to our own "OCD" or "ADD," deemed a mercurial sibling "seriously bipolar," written off an erratic ex as "obviously borderline," or nodded as a laid-off friend pronounced his former boss a "textbook sociopath"?

Lately, a new kind of head case stalks the land—staring past us, blurting gaucheries, droning on about the technical minutiae of his boring hobby. And we are ready with our *DSM* codes: 299.00 (autistic disorder) and 299.80 (Asperger's disorder).

The pros have led the way. In the nineties, clinicians began reconceptualizing autism from a singular disorder to a cluster of related conditions on a spectrum of severity; as the criteria broadened to encompass less acutely impaired people—such as the more verbal group diagnosed with Asperger's—prevalence rose dramatically. Before 1980, one in 2,000 children was thought to be autistic. By 2007, the Centers for Disease Control were reporting that one in 152 American children had an autism spectrum disorder. Two years later, the CDC updated the ratio to one in 110. This past March, the CDC revised the number upward again, to one in 88 (one in 54, if you just count boys, who are five times as likely to have one as girls). A South Korean study from last year put the number even higher, at one in 38. And in New Jersey, according to the latest numbers, an improbable one in 29 boys is on the spectrum.

Despite much debate about the causes of the so-called autism epidemic, the consensus among experts is that the increase is mostly due not to a rise in incidence but to greater awareness, recognition, and testing, and to the wider parameters of who qualifies for a place on the spectrum (New Jersey, for instance, has some of the most robust autism services in the country). Such elasticity is nowhere so relevant as at the fuzzy, ever-shifting threshold where clinical disorder shades into everyday eccentricity. The upper end of the spectrum is the liminal zone where Aspies, as people with Asperger's call themselves, reside.

But this is not a story about Asperger's, autism, or the spectrum—those very real afflictions that can bring untold hardship to the people who suffer from them and to their families. It is, instead, a story about "Asperger's," "autism," and "the spectrum"—our one-stop-shopping shorthand for the jerky husband, the socially inept plutocrat, the tactless boss, the child prodigy with no friends, the remorseless criminal. It's about the words we deploy to describe some murky hybrid of egghead and aloof.

Like the actual clinical disorder, the cultural epidemic in scare quotes may have less to do with changes in the world than with changes in those seeing it. To some degree, the spectrum is our way of making sense of an upended social topography, a buckled landscape where nerd titans hold the high ground once occupied by square-jawed captains of industry, a befuddling digital world overrun with trolls and avatars and social-media "rock stars" who are nothing like actual rock stars. It is, as the amateur presidential shrinks would have it, a handy phrase for the distant, cerebral men with the ambition and self-possession necessary to mount a serious run for the White House. When quants and engineers are ascendant, when algorithms trump the liberal arts, when Kim Kardashian and Justin Bieber tweet about the death of Steve Jobs, when the hyperspecialist has displaced the generalist and everyone is *Matrix*-ed into the Internet, it's an Other-deriding tool to soothe our cultural anxiety about the ongoing power shift from humanists to technologists. As the coders inherit the Earth, saying someone's on the spectrum is how English majors make themselves feel better.

But anxiety alone (generalized anxiety disorder: 300.02) doesn't fully explain it. There's something admiring, too, in the cultural uses of Asperger's, which makes it different from the psych put-downs du jour of previous eras. The popular but mostly false image of *Rain Man*-like asocial geniuses (whether on the sitcoms *Big Bang Theory* and *Community,* say, or in best-selling books like Jodi Picoult's novel *House Rules* and Michael Lewis's *The Big Short*) has helped create a mystique around high-functioning autism, and the idea that Asperger's offers selective advantages has midwifed a generation of self-outers: See, for example, Pulitzer Prize-winning music critic Tim Page's *Parallel Play: Growing Up With Undiagnosed Asperger's,* or contestant Heather Kuzmich's appearances on *America's Next Top Model.*

And so we find ourselves in a weird place. A psychiatric diagnosis first observed in four boys more than half a century ago has become common slang, a conceptual gadget for processing the modern world. Weirder still: At the same time it soothes the insecurities of those who would weaponize it as insult, it flatters the vanity of those who'd appropriate it as status credential.

In 1995, when Ben Nugent was 17 years old, his mother told him she thought he had Asperger's. This was particularly distressing to him, both because his mother was qualified to know—she was a psychologist specializing in the disorder—and because he was an aspiring novelist. As he puts it: "If what I had proposed to do with my life was to plumb the inner depths of other people, it could be a big problem." He never actually believed he had Asperger's, but at the time, it hadn't yet become a pop-culture phenomenon, and when his mother asked him to appear in an educational video she was making about the disorder, he agreed. By the time he watched the film for the first time, he was 22, lived in New York, worked as an arts reporter at *Time,* and had a new set of friends, and it was clear to him that he was neurologically typical. His girlfriend laughed as they watched the video together and he kept objecting to his inclusion. "When I saw this video and saw what the other people in it were like," Nugent says, "I was like, *Oh my God.*"

"I was totally awkward," Nugent says of his younger years, "but awkward in a totally normal way. I was an aspiring hipster in a bad vintage polo shirt and a Blur haircut talking about the understanding of literature I had in fifth grade. So, really annoying probably, but not on the autism spectrum."

Other than several years' resentment toward his mother, who was profusely apologetic, and free ammo for opponents ("A girlfriend who wanted to win an argument would say, 'Maybe your mom was right' "), Nugent seems to have survived the episode unscathed, and he's become something of a student of the modern conflation of social awkwardness with autism. In his nonfiction *American Nerd: The Story of My People,* he included a chart that matched up the diagnostic criteria for Asperger's with a list of classic nerd traits (social phobias, rule-bound speech, etc.). "If you look at certain nerd characters, like Jerry Lewis in *The Nutty Professor,*" Nugent says, "he's basically acting like someone with Asperger's or mild autism. He's spastic, doesn't understand social cues, is a savant." More recently, Nugent wrote an op-ed in the *Times* lamenting the overdiagnosis of Asperger's.

Not that Nugent himself is always rigorous in applying the label to others. "When I get mad at someone I have a retail interaction with, like if I'm attempting to buy a shirt from someone who doesn't understand what I'm saying, later I'll say, 'That guy was kind of Asperger's-y.' It means: not sensitive to my needs. I'm guilty of using the term in a sloppy vernacular way like everyone else."

The vagueness of the border between able and disabled has made Asperger's controversial from the time it was coined as a diagnosis, in 1981, by English psychiatrist Lorna Wing. Wing named it after Hans Asperger, a Viennese pediatrician who in a 1944 paper had described four boys as sharing "a lack of empathy, little ability to form friendships, one-sided conversations, intense absorption in a special interest, and clumsy movements." He called them "little professors." (Asperger himself seems to have been a bit spectrum-y as a child, endlessly reciting the verse of Austrian poet Franz Grillparzer, to his classmates' dismay.) By 1990, Asperger's syndrome was in common usage among clinicians as a term to describe a distinct verbal subset of autistics.

But exactly how Asperger's made it into the *DSM-IV,* published in 1994, remains veiled in mystery.

The history of psychiatry is a long fade-in, a glacial zoom toward granularity. Autism emerged from a conceptual catchall called "childhood schizophrenia," and Asperger's, in turn, was carved out of autism. But the more fine-grained the distinctions, the more they threaten to overlap and blur into each other. The community of clinicians specializing in developmental neurologys generally viewed *DSM-IIIR,* which had been published in 1987, as wildly overinclusive. It had only two categories of spectrum disorders—autism and the kitchen-sink PDD-NOS (pervasive developmental disorder-not otherwise specified)—and its imprecision was seen as having led to an alarming increase in the number of diagnoses.

The overarching agenda of *DSM-IV,* then, was to be more specific and to raise the bar for diagnosis. By the early nineties, the committee tasked with revising the taxonomy was focusing on whether Asperger's was fundamentally different from high-functioning autism. But their work was conscribed to hashing out the pros and cons of creating a separate diagnosis for Asperger's and didn't extend to making a decision or establishing what the diagnostic criteria would be. That work would fall to nonspecialist higher-ups at the APA. Even as the committee finished several years' work, its members had no idea whether Asperger's would make it into the big book. "It was like the election of the pope," says Peter Szatmari, a leading Canadian researcher who sat on the working group. "The message went upstairs, and we waited around for smoke to come out of the Vatican. And there it was."

The science writers hired to draft the *DSM-IV* text inexplicably dropped one of the criteria the committee had agreed distinguished Asperger's: gross motor clumsiness. And, arbitrarily, they decided that the criteria for Asperger's would be the same as for autism, with simply a different number of criteria needing to be met to qualify. "Asperger's got put in at the last minute," recalls working-group chairman Fred Volkmar, head of child psychiatry at the Yale–New Haven Children's Hospital, "with a lot of tweaking of it by powers on high ... There's so much of a rush to get the finished book done and copyedited and out. Things happen." Volkmar says that for the PDD-NOS diagnosis, a copy editor who happened not to like an "and" replaced it with "or," a seemingly tiny change that significantly expanded the diagnosis.

The publication of *DSM-IV* had unintended consequences. "We were glad that Asperger's was included," says psychologist Bryna Siegel, another working-group member, who directs clinical care at the autism clinic at the University of California, San Francisco, "but until the publication of *DSM-IV*, very few people had heard the term *Asperger's*. And when it came out, a lot of clinicians let their fingers do the walking in *DSM*. There were fully trained practicing clinicians who really didn't have any idea what Asperger's was. Everybody with Asperger's got diagnosed with Asperger's, but a lot of other people got diagnosed with Asperger's, too."

Siegel, who has been running her clinic since the eighties, says she's seeing "more false-positive assessments than ever before." Of the roughly ten new assessments she's asked to do every week—kids showing up with spectrum diagnoses from another therapist—six of them might not have an autism-spectrum disorder. This isn't to say that they may not have psychological issues, only that those are either other disorders or they don't rise to an impairing level. "A lot of kids are just delayed in development, slow to talk, or anxious, or hyperactive, and a lot of kids are just terribly parented."

Siegel sees overdiagnosis and misdiagnosis as driven largely by economic and social priorities rather than medical ones. Some adults who might be very high-functioning seek a formal diagnosis because it enables them to, in Siegel's words, "wallow" in their symptoms rather than "ameliorate" them, because they're "a lunch ticket." Poor parents want diagnoses serious enough to merit state-funded school services, and rich parents want the least stigmatizing diagnoses. ("When you say a kid is mentally retarded," Siegel says, "parents try to talk you out of it.") And some parents are simply flummoxed by their own kids' irrational mood swings, refusal of food, or inability to express emotion. When these parents come to Siegel, they get a surprise: She diagnoses their children as suffering from childhood. "We see a lot of diagnosis-of-childhood kids, whose parents have never set limits, plus kids who are temperamentally difficult to raise."

Also temperamentally difficult: husbands. Put-upon spouses have seized on the autism rainbow as a simple, esteem-boosting way to pathologize what used to be called "a typical guy." Simon Baron-Cohen, a leading expert on Asperger's at Cambridge (and, as it happens, the cousin of Sacha), has theorized that the autism spectrum represents the "extreme male brain," turned up to eleven. Hence the ubiquity of spectrum references in the coastal power centers where Nora Ephron spent most of her time. And the Internet abounds with unhappy married women diagnosing their callous workaholic husbands with Asperger's, whether or not a clinician has seconded their opinion. In a forum called Asperger Divorce Support Group, posters share war stories, some less harrowing than others: "My ex ... did not GET a sunset. He took pictures of fall color trees last year and said, 'I guess it's cool looking, right?' "

"It's become more frequent in the last five years," confirms a Connecticut divorce lawyer who says she has represented parties in several cases where a wife accused the husband of being on the spectrum. "It's women complaining, 'He lines up my towels perfectly. He complains if his shoes aren't lined up right.' "

Men have caught on and, in a kind of inverted gaslighting, begun to describe themselves as having Asperger's as a way of controlling their spouses. "Having Asperger's-like syndrome does not give you Asperger's," says David Schnarch, a Colorado-based couples therapist. "Having a big belly does not make you pregnant. I've not seen a single case of what I would consider to be diagnosable Asperger's. But I have seen any number of cases of wives accusing husbands of it, any number of cases of husbands claiming to have it." It's the new ADHD, he says. "The wife doesn't want to accept that the husband knows what he's doing when he's doing something she doesn't like." Schnarch recalls a man who phoned him the day before a scheduled initial couples session and announced that he'd just been diagnosed with Asperger's. "As soon as this happened," Schnarch says, "I knew I had difficulty." He contacted the referring therapist, who said he'd suspected the man had Asperger's because he said things to his girlfriend that were so cruel he couldn't possibly understand their impact. As far as Schnarch was concerned, it was an all-too-familiar instance of sadism masquerading as disability. "If you're going to perp, the best place to perp from is the victim position."

Because Asperger's lives on the outskirts of normal, and because its symptoms can resemble willfully antisocial behavior, there's now a presumption of excuse-making whenever someone invokes it to get out of a pickle. Last October, *South Park* aired an episode in which the people at an Asperger's group-therapy center turn out to be faking their symptoms and not even to believe in the reality of the disorder. (Cartman, meanwhile, mishearing Asperger's as "Ass Burgers," tries to fake it by stuffing his underwear with hamburgers.) "You're not autistic," a doctor tells Hugh Laurie's abrasive character in an episode of *House*. "You don't even have Asperger's. You wish you did; it would exempt you from the rules, give you freedom, absolve you of responsibility, let you date 17-year-olds. But, most important, it would mean that you're not just a jerk."

The yen to see the world in SpectrumVision is not just a case of glib metaphor abuse. Some studies of twins suggest that autism traits are distributed throughout the population. And it's now understood that there's an autism phenotype, where the same genetics can manifest in mild forms in parents and as full-blown autism in their children.

No one has been so responsible for the spread of this idea as Baron-Cohen, who has conducted a number of studies showing concentrations of autism among techies. In 1997, he published one asserting that autistic children were twice as likely as non-autistic children to have fathers or grandfathers who were engineers; he found a higher rate of autistic traits among math students at Cambridge than among those in other disciplines; and he has argued that in Silicon Valley, geeks intermarry and are more likely to produce autistic offspring.

As it turns out, a striking number of criminal defendants diagnosed with Asperger's are computer hackers. Misha Glenny, author of a book about cybercrime, is convinced that hackers are often people on the spectrum who end up outside the law by default—their lack of social skills combined with a surplus of computer know-how. "The Internet is what has made them—it gave them a place to be criminals," he has said. Earlier this month, the British home secretary ruled against the extradition to the U.S. of Gary McKinnon, a hacker who in 2002 was arrested for breaking into dozens of American government computers in what a U.S. attorney called "the biggest hack of military computers ever." McKinnon, who has been diagnosed with Asperger's, has said that he was just trying to unearth proof that the government was covering up UFO secrets, including anti-gravity technology acquired from alien landings. He has become a cause célèbre, inspiring Free Gary T-shirts and a benefit song featuring Chrissie Hynde, Bob Geldof, and David Gilmour. McKinnon's diagnosis dates only to 2008, after a television viewer with Asperger's saw a news report about the case and contacted McKinnon's lawyer, who then had McKinnon evaluated by Baron-Cohen.

Baron-Cohen has come in for criticism by scholars and some autism advocates who view his methods as unrigorous. Other researchers have pointed out that so-called autism clusters tend to be in areas with more highly educated people—who tend to marry older (a factor that correlates with higher autism rates) and who have the money to have their kids tested. "I don't think Baron-Cohen understands the rudiments of genetics," says Jonathan Mitchell, a high-functioning autistic who writes the Autism's Gadfly blog. But Baron-Cohen's work gets all the media play. In 2001, *Wired* published an article, "The Geek Syndrome," popularizing the autistic-nerd meme. It was accompanied by Baron-Cohen's 50-question self-diagnostic questionnaire, and afterward, says Bryna Siegel, whose clinic is a short drive from Silicon Valley, "we had an incredible number of phone calls. I told my assistant, 'If someone has their secretary call, don't call back. If they have a secretary, they don't have Asperger's.' "

The self-diagnosis boom has been accompanied by self-diagnoses that can be bracing in their unpersuasiveness. Craigslist's Newmark has acknowledged that "psychologist friends" have dismissed his self-diagnosis as "hypochondria." Bram Cohen, the founder of BitTorrent, has revealed that his self-professed Asperger's, about which he has spoken publicly at great length, was suggested by his girlfriend and never confirmed by a professional. Nobel Prize-winning economist Vernon Smith, another self-diagnoser, has cited as a key symptom the "tremendous amount of strain" he finds in "a social situation that lasts a couple of hours."

Aspies, self-diagnosed and otherwise, speak of the relief that diagnosis brings. For someone who may have gone decades feeling socially alienated, and blaming himself for it, knowledge of the condition can offer a key to the puzzle of his personality and the interpersonal challenges he's experienced. It was "a biblical weight off," and an explanation "for all those social banana peels along the way," says Michael John Carley, who was diagnosed at 36, after his 4-year-old son was diagnosed with Asperger's.

Carley has an unusual background for someone with a disorder characterized by difficulty in social interaction; a graduate of Columbia, he previously worked as a diplomat in Bosnia and Iraq. He is now a leading Asperger's advocate, one of a vocal group who promote the idea of "neurodiversity" and consider non-autistic people to be "neurotypicals," or "NTs," with different but not superior cognitive styles.

The Aspie-pride movement—an extreme fringe of which goes so far as to argue for "autistic supremacy"—takes its intellectual framework partly from studies that have posited that autism is an evolutionary adaptation, enabling survival strategies including solitary foraging, and that a male in the ancestral environment might have benefited from being more systematic and less empathic than others. Penny Spikins, an archaeologist at the University of York, recently published a paper suggesting that autistics were responsible for nothing less than the Stone Age tool revolution. Others, such as Juan Enriquez, a "futurist" at Harvard Business School, have argued that autism isn't so much a vestige of the past as a glimpse of what's to come: "the next evolutionary step" in an increasingly data-choked world.

Less grandly, there may be something to the idea of an affinity between autistics and the Information Age, given that autistics, with their difficulty imagining minds apart from their own, tend to relate better to animals and machines than to people. Online, the off-putting physical manifestations of spectrum disorders are stripped away. Celebrity autistic Temple Grandin has said that "there is nothing out there closer to how I think" than the web, with its structure of associative links. The web is shaping our behavior in "what is broadly a more autistic direction," argues behavioral economist Tyler Cowen, such as the way it lets us "pursue our identities and alliances based around very specific and articulable interests." (Mobile phones, too: In the utilitarian, no-small-talk idiom of texting, he sees an autistic style of communication.)

The investor Peter Thiel has said of Internet companies that "the people who run them are sort of autistic. These mild cases of Asperger's seem to be quite rampant. There's no need for sales—the companies themselves are weirdly nonsocial in nature." This is a vision of Internet culture as spectral, of whole corporations that miss social cues. It explains how services like Facebook and Google continually offend people with their missteps—whether changing privacy settings without permission, or photographing homes for Google Earth, or, in the case of businesses like Napster and BitTorrent, being completely indifferent to intellectual property—and then seem genuinely, naïvely surprised.

Still, it has become fashionable in some circles to describe the spectrum as the very womb of modernity. "If you were to get rid of all the autism genetics, there would be no more Silicon Valley," Grandin told a ted audience. David Mamet, in his book *Bambi vs. Godzilla,* writes, "I think it is not impossible that Asperger's syndrome helped make the movies," citing such movie-director traits as "early precocity," high information-processing capacity, attachment to routine, unconventionality, and social deficits. A recent ripple of business journalism has emphasized the narrow competencies of those on the high-functioning end of the spectrum as a competitive advantage: "In Praise of Misfits" (*The Economist*), "If You Really Want to Innovate, Put an Autistic

Person on Your Team" (*Business Insider*). Specialisterne, a Danish company, employs 60 people on the spectrum to do software testing and other repetitive tasks.

Cowen, one of the most prominent champions of autism-as-superpower, came to believe he has "an autistic cognitive style" after receiving an e-mail suggesting as much from a reader of his blog, and has credited his take on autism as being "much influenced" by his former colleague Vernon Smith. In *The Age of the Infovore,* Cowen makes the energetic if labored case that autism is "a hidden cultural force" and that "understanding human neurodiversity in terms of impairments is fundamentally misleading." He extols autistics' "cognitive strengths": "They are better at noticing details in patterns, they have better eyesight on average, they are less likely to be fooled by optical illusions ... and they are less likely to have false memories of particular kinds." In his zeal to present autism in a positive light, Cowen flirts with dottiness, writing things like, "Autistics are the culmination of Buddhist thought and indeed Buddhist practice," and coming very close to diagnosing the entire country of Finland as autistic.

The same rose-colored impulse has driven an Aspie wave of revisionist psychopathography, in which such diverse historical figures as Thomas Jefferson, Orson Welles, Charles Darwin, Albert Einstein, Isaac Newton, Andy Warhol, and Wolfgang Amadeus Mozart are supposed to have been residents of the spectrum. The time-traveling diagnoses often feel like cloud-reading—the case for Darwin as Aspie, as set forth in *Genius Genes: How Asperger Talents Changed the World,* relies on diagnostic bullet points: his childhood as "something of a loner," his "obsession" with nature, his routine of counting the laps of his nightly walks in later life. They also seem to have fueled more diagnoses in the present. "I got a letter from around the world from a man who was diagnosed when he was 80," says *Genius Genes* co-author Michael Fitzgerald, a professor of child psychiatry at

Trinity College, Dublin. "A lot of people read my book, and that was the first time they found they had autism. Someone rang me from China to say he'd read about his distant relative in the Civil War and for the first time realized he had Asperger's."

Even fictional characters come in for the treatment. In 2008, the *Journal of Positive Behavior Interventions* published a peer-reviewed article about "nonconforming, socially awkward" Bartleby the Scrivener, arguing that "retrospective analysis indicates that Bartleby may in fact have been a victim of the modern diagnosis of autism spectrum disorder, more specifically, a high-functioning form of autism termed Asperger's syndrome." Cowen, for his part, avers in *Infovore* that Sherlock Holmes is "the most fully developed autistic character in the Western literary tradition."

For clinicians in the trenches, the more exuberant efforts to link autism with genius can be exasperating. "Do blind people hear music more exquisitely than people with sight?" asks Siegel. "We don't have any neurophysiological evidence that they do." Similarly, most people with Asperger's have average intelligence, with high IQs the exception. And many with ASD, and the families who care for them, suffer terribly. "There clearly are people with ASD who marry," says Catherine Lord, director of the Center for Autism and the Developing Brain at Weill Cornell Medical College, "but they are not many. More and more people with ASD have jobs, but the majority are underemployed, or have jobs that don't use their capabilities as much as possible. So these references to Einstein and Jefferson are not helpful."

At 6 p.m. on a recent Wednesday, in a carpeted rent-by-the-hour room in a sixteenth-floor conference center near Penn Station, some 25 people have gathered for the monthly meeting of a Manhattan Asperger's support group.

It's a largely male, mostly white group, ranging from a teenager to people in their sixties. They seem afflicted, or visibly off, to different degrees. Some appear to be straight-up NTs. Some, shorts hiked high, look like central-casting nerds. A handful have strange affects: A young Orthodox Jewish man in his late twenties smiles to himself, and another young man holds his hands near his chest, silent and fidgeting. Many, though, are smiling and socializing. "I like your forest shirt," one man says to a taciturn man named Gabe, who wears a green polo shirt patterned with trees.

Karl, a former engineer who runs the group for the Global Regional Asperger Syndrome Partnership (grasp), begins the meeting by having everyone in the room introduce himself: first name, diagnosis, employment and relationship status. As they speak, Karl chimes in occasionally, speaking in a distinctly enunciated, arrhythmic way. For a lot of the people here, Asperger's isn't their only problem. "Autism, borderline-personality disorder, depression, diabetes," one person says. Another person says: "1997, self-diagnosed; 1998, clinically diagnosed." A graphic designer named David got an online diagnosis after his six-and-a-half-year marriage crumbled: "My husband always said I had something." Nearly everyone is single, and a good number live with their parents.

A British woman, talking about a popular Asperger's memoir, John Elder Robison's *Look Me in the Eye,* starts crying, saying what a relief it had been to read, flooding her with memories of her own experiences; she'd always thought she was "daft." The room fills with a chorus of sympathetic voices ("It's okay to cry," another woman reassures her). These don't look like people seeking an excuse, or imagining a set of problems, or lacking in feeling, or just being eccentric. They seem to see the world through a particular lens, to have significant if narrow competencies, to be really struggling.

And their world is about to get shaken up. Next May, the fifth edition of the *DSM* is to be published, and the APA has proposed to eliminate the Asperger's diagnosis, folding it, as well as PDD-NOS, into the broader new all-purpose bucket of autism spectrum disorder. The thinking is that Asperger's isn't scientifically distinguishable from autism, and that a single diagnosis may help to combat the epidemic that is more diagnostic than real. But the debate has been fractious. Fred Volkmar, who'd headed the committee for *DSM-IV,* quit the *DSM-5* committee, and has been vocal about the likelihood that the redrawn map of who's on the spectrum will cause a lot of people who currently have diagnoses to lose them. A report previewed in January suggested that as few as 45 percent of people who currently have Asperger's or PDD-NOS diagnoses will retain them, though a study in *The American Journal of Psychiatry,* published earlier this month, put the number closer to 90 percent.

For the people in this room, Asperger's is an identity as much as a diagnosis, and as much as this is a specialists' debate with real-world implications (insurance, school services), it's also an existential koan: If you lose your Asperger's diagnosis, do you not have Asperger's? Did you ever? grasp will continue to exist, but Karl tells the room that the AS may change to standing for Autism Spectrum, and Michael Carley, the head of grasp, has written a book titled *The Last Memoir of Asperger's Syndrome.* "I think I would say, if the term Asperger's helps you describe yourself and gives you community, use it," Catherine Lord, who is on the *DSM-5* committee, tells me. "The fact that we're changing the medical diagnosis ... Most people who use Asperger's would not have met the *DSM-IV* criteria, so they're using the term already as a colloquial term. And that's fine. I don't think anyone wants to take that away, it just isn't a medical diagnosis. If someone needs someone to cut them slack, whether they have Asperger's or not, that's something they need to negotiate with their spouse."

Among the members of tonight's support group, people fall on both sides of the debate. "My belief," says an older man named Allen, "is it's impossible to distinguish Asperger's from high-functioning autism. It has more to do with where you get a diagnosis than the scientific criteria."

"What will it do for people who already have a diagnosis?" Gabe, in the green forest shirt, asks. "Where will we be? Anybody who agrees with me that Asperger's shouldn't be clumped under ASD, say 'No.' "

There are lots of "No"s. Someone mentions that the New York State Assembly is considering passing a law to exempt the state from the *DSM-5*.

"Yes!" Gabe says, doing a closed-fist power salute. "We can't just throw up our hands. What about Aspies and generations to come?"

"Woody Allen still makes movies about neurotics," Allen points out.

"Let's keep calling ourselves Aspies," Gabe says.

"Oh, hellz yes," says a guy in back.

SECTION V

SUMMATION

TRIBUTE TO MOM & DAD by Jon Wallace

MOM

Mom, thanks for being my link to God. You have anchored me in him/her. You have always been inspired by God and have had a close connection to him/her. You influenced me to have the desire to come close to God. God is the source of all life, prosperity, and victory, so I want to thank you for what you have done for me. How you have brought me closer to God.

Like God is my divine mother, you are too, Mom. You exercise those loving, nurturing, compassionate, giving qualities. I love you as you have loved me so much. You have always been there for me, to support me in a number of ways including emotionally. You have been there through my ups and my downs with tender love and care. You have propelled me forward to be a strong individual. You have corrected me when I've been wrong, including morally. Because of you I am a better person. I have learned to be more loving, joyful, kind, and more. You have been a living example of these qualities yourself. I have seen this when you have given some money to a homeless person. When you have spoken some words of kindness and encouragement to someone. I have seen this in the way you honor your relationships with your friends. The way you have been there to help them through tough times and celebrate their good times just as you have with me.

You also have done this for Dad as well. A lot of the time you have been there for Dad in the way of pushing him forward. You become really concerned and push him to make a difference within himself. I know you do this because you care about him, just as you have cared for me. Thank you so much, Mom, for being such a blessing of love, joy, kindness, giving, caring, and compassion, for displaying this so much with me, Dad, all of your family, and friends. Also, even with people in general that you come across daily.

I love you infinitely, Mom. With my hands connected and extended behind my back, I love you this Much!!! (inside joke). You are divinity in motion. You are a divine expression of God. You are a joy-felt teardrop of His. You are the rising of the sun. You are the moon and stars in the sky. You are full of purity as is the beautiful dove. You are angelic. You are an angel. I wish you more peace, prosperity, and many more blessings. More blessings than you can count. Thank you for everything, Mom, I love you.

DAD

Dad, as God is my heavenly father my provider, you are my provider as well. Thanks for providing me and supporting me throughout my life in a numerous amount of ways. Thank you for supporting me financially. You have always given me a beautiful house to live in, a luxurious bed to sleep in, water to drink, food on the table to eat, and all other kinds of amenities. You have given me amenities that are necessities and ones that are non-necessities, just very extraordinary. Thank you for your immense, amazing, tireless, work of which you have partaken in to support our family financially. You sacrifice yourself and push yourself in a grueling way to be able to give to our family abundantly. You are very much so appreciated for that. I would like to see you be easier on yourself. I do appreciate your intense efforts, though. I know that Mom does, too. We thank you.

Thank you for your common sense, of which I in the past have much lacked. I have decided to listen to you more now, so that I can be grounded in sense and have common sense myself.

Thank you for your words of wisdom as well, too. You speak many of them, and coming from experience. Thank you, Dad.

Dad you are our golden warrior, our Rocky Balboa. You're strong, a champ. You fight a fight so we don't have to. We can most of the time lay back and take it easy. Once again, you also provide us with wisdom, the wisdom of a wise man. With this fundamental, we are more grounded and stable as a family. Thank you, Dad, I look forward to learning a lot more from you. Thank you for everything. I love you, infinitely.

MY JOURNEY by Ann Hamilton Wallace

How is it possible to summarize a journey such as this one? I don't know. I think I will write from the heart. I will think of all of you as a best friend that I want to guide through the process.

Some couples say they are "childless by choice"; in other words, they don't want the pressure or bother of raising ungrateful monsters. They say that's all they see nowadays. I say it's poor parenting and not setting limits. That's why I am stressing to you: don't use the autistic label to promote bad behavior. It's very important to teach your youngsters social skills, which will serve them as they grow.

Jon is loved by young and old. The 3 year old in our building looks forward to doing the twist with our son and laughing all the way. The seniors at the Villa Sunrise, where my mom lives, all ask if my wonderful son is coming with me to visit. (They miss him.) One of my best friends tells me she wished Jon would wait to marry her 14-year-old daughter. My friend knows Jon from the time he was 5 years old, knows he's autistic, and doesn't give it any consideration.

"I love him," she says. "He is the kindest, most wonderful kid I know."

Putting that all aside, is life with Jon a total breeze? No. If I want him to rush because we are late, he slows down.

If I want a commitment from him, he won't commit.

He checks the windows and doors so much for security at night, he has broken the handles off. Then, there are the misunderstandings about the point I'm trying to make, which start numerous arguments. And he will leave our conversations midstream to go to his "quiet room" to decompress. But there's always that great smile and apology that warms my heart.

I'm living with an eccentric, warm-hearted son that loves me to death. And I love him beyond what words can express.

He is so talented and creative it blows my mind. And there's never a dull moment in our home. When he was diagnosed so many years ago by B.J. Freeman at UCLA, she did not give us much hope.

"He won't finish high school (it's too abstract for him)," she said, adding he won't drive, he won't marry. "The good news is he is not retarded."

At that point, I couldn't hear anything good about her prognosis. My friends, don't be discouraged. Expert or not, she was wrong! Jon has been able to achieve on a level with all the "neurotypicals" out there. He finished high school with good grades and gets abstract concepts with the best of them. His driving abilities are superior; he has never had an accident even though my friends' "neurotypicals" have smashed their cars several times, to their mothers' and insurance carriers' dismay.

As far as a wife, I believe that is to come. When the right girl shows up, a wedding will surely follow.

The point of this is: never be told "bad news." Always take things day by day and be optimistic about you and your child.*+

As Dr. Ricki Robinson said, "Don't have ceilings in place; learning is a lifelong process."

And remember Dr. Wallace said not to try to push a square peg into a round hole. Don't go the typical college route if that is not your child's desire or interest. Happiness is everything and should be the goal. A happy child is a blessing for the both of you.

Now, go do the right thing, and I know you will!

Jon's Song by Arlene Artale

Could he have been a river?
He did seem to flow free.
And though he had a way to go
He moved effortlessly.

So deep in place he couldn't see,
He knew it just the same.
And like a river skimmed the stones,
As if they were his claim.

Rivers they need to keep moving,
and spreading their reach into streams.
Don't you know if he had to stay in one place,
There's no way that he could reach his dreams?

But maybe he was a flower,
With petals translucent and light,
That burst from a pod ripe with passion,
And reaching for all that is right.

As he swayed with the breeze he kept tandem,
Though he would have preferred to move free.
But he didn't want to break at the stem,
After all, he wasn't a tree.

Flowers are objects of beauty;
With their colors and fragrance and such.
And they remind me so much of him
Just like him they enhance all they touch.

No, I'm sure that he was a rainbow, and all of us just didn't know.
As he beamed such beautiful colors,
And gave us a mystical show.

One moment he would be here,
And then so far away.
Then like a rainbow reappeared,
And gently graced the day.

Rainbows are only illusions.
That's likely the reason why –
He always seemed too bright for here,
His true place was ever so high.

Divine Romance by Jon Wallace

I was in the pit of hell.

Like a phoenix, I arose from the ashes
and I am now ascending to my ultimate destination,
the celestial heavenly realms of you.

There I will unite with you
and partake in a divine cosmic romantic dance with you.
I will drink from thy immortal cup of life
and let thy wine of life pulsate and flow through my heart,
entire mind-body complex and inner soul kingdom,
recharging every atom of my being with the elixir of your divine
love, light and bliss.

I will be a wave united with your pure, warm, pristine ocean of love.
Your passionate fire of divine love will burn deep within me
disintegrating the negative karma seed and roots in me.

Through my labor of love we together will plant within me posi-
tive seeds
and I will reap abundant, delicious fruit
of which I will eat plentifully and let the juices drip down my chin.
At last, dear God I am one with you, my divine romance.

My beloved God, thank you, I love you.

AFTERWORD

Always reach, strive, climb, and find the life that awaits you. Never compare your child to another. Everyone's journey is an individual's challenge against personal goals and desires. Happiness is the victor, my son Jon often reminds me. Happiness is a choice. We chose happiness.

AHW

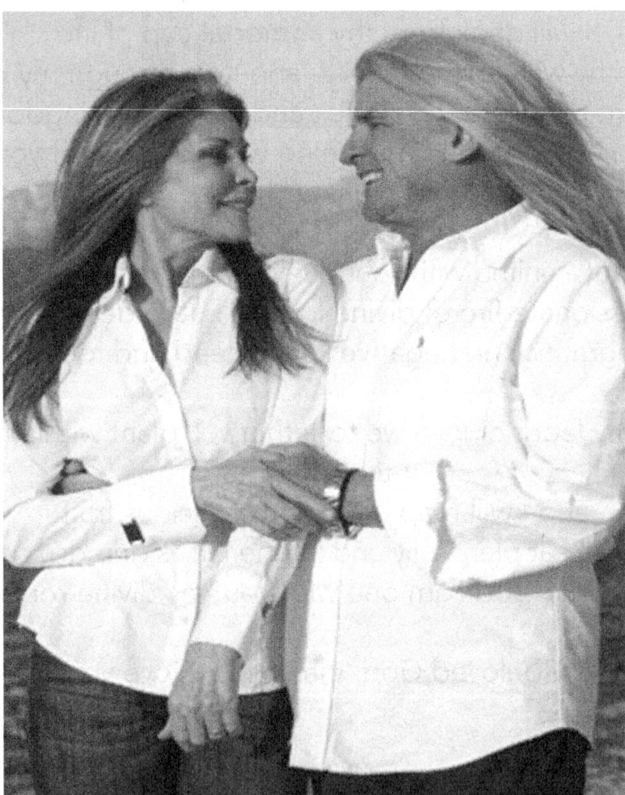

SUGGESTED READING LIST

A Mind at a Time: America's Top Learning Expert Shows How Every Child Can Succeed, Mel Levine, M.D., Simon & Schuster, New York, 2002.

Asperger's Syndrome: A Guide for Parents and Professionals, Tony Atwood, Jessica Kingsley Publishers, London and Philadelphia, 1998.

Autism Solutions: How to Create a Healthy and Meaningful Life for Your Child, Ricki G. Robinson, M.D., M.P.H., Harlequin, Ontario, Canada, 2011.

Between Their World and Ours: Breakthrough with Autistic Children, Karen Zelan, St. Martin's Griffin, 2004.

The Brain's Way of Healing: Remarkable Discoveries and Recoveries from the Frontiers of Neuroplasticity, Norman Doidge, M.D., Penguin Group, New York, 2015

Callous Disregard: Autism and Vaccines: The Truth Behind a Tragedy, Andrew J Wakefield, Skyhorse Publishing, New York, 2010.

Day by Day: Raising the Child with Autism/PDD, Joan F. Goodman and Susan Hoban, Guilford Publications (video & manual), New York, 1992.

Diet for a New America: How Your Food Choices Affect Your Health, Happiness and the Future of Life on Earth, John Robbins, HJ Kramer/New World Library, 25th Anniversary Edition, 2012.

Diet Intervention and Autism: Implementing the Gluten Free and Casein Free Diet for Autistic Children and Adults: A Practical Guide for Parents, Marilyn Le Breton, Jessica Kingsley Publishers, London and Philadelphia, 2001.

The Game of My Life: A True Story of Challenge, Triumph, and Growing Up Autistic, Jason "J-Mac" McElwain with Daniel Paisner, New American Library, New York, 2008.

Gut and Psychology Syndrome: Natural Treatment for Autism, Dyspraxia, A.D.D., Dyslexia, A.D.H.D., Depression, Schizophrenia (GAPS Diet), Natasha Campbell-McBride, Medinform Publishing, 2010.

Healing and Preventing Autism: A Complete Guide, Jenny McCarthy and Jerry Kartzinel, M.D., Dutton, Penguin Group, New York, 2009.

High-Functioning Individuals with Autism, Eric Schopler and Gary B. Mesibov, Plenum Press, New York and London, 1992.

Learning Disabilities and Social Skills with Richard Lavoie: A Teacher's Guide, Last One Picked . . . First One Picked On, Richard Lavoie, PBS Video, 1994.

Let Me Hear Your Voice: A Family's Triumph Over Autism, Catherine Maurice, The Random House Publishing Group, 1994.

Say Good-Bye to Allergy-Related Autism, Devi S. Nambudripad, Delta Publishing Co., 1999.

Six-Word Lessons on Growing Up Autistic: 100 Lessons to Understand How Autistic People See Life, Trevor Pacelli, Leading on the Edge International, Bellevue, Washington, 2012.

Solve Your Child's Sleep Problems, Richard Ferber, M.D., Fireside/ Simon & Schuster, Inc. New York, 1985, 2006.

Teaching Individuals with Developmental Delays, O. Ivar Lovaas, Pro ed, 2002.

Through the Eyes of Aliens: A Book About Autistic People, Jasmine Lee O'Neill, Jessica Kingsley Publishers, Ltd., London and Philadelphia, 1999.

When the Brain Can't Hear: Unraveling the Mystery of Auditory Processing Disorder, Terri James Bellis, Ph.D., Atria Books, New York, 2003.

When Slow Is Fast Enough: Educating the Delayed Preschool Child, Joan F. Goodman, The Guilford Press, New York and London, 1992.

The World of the Autistic Child: Understanding and Treating Autistic Spectrum Disorders, Bryna Siegel, Ph.D., Oxford University Press, Inc., 1998.

INDEX

B

C

D

E

F

G

H

N

O

P

Q

R

S